Kava

Medicinal and Aromatic Plants – Industrial Profiles

Individual volumes in this series provide both industry and academia with in-depth coverage of one major genus of industrial importance.

Edited by Dr Roland Hardman

Volume 1
Valerian, edited by Peter J. Houghton

Volume 2
Perilla, edited by He-ci Yu, Kenichi Kosuna and Megumi Haga

Volume 3
Poppy, edited by Jenö Bernáth

Volume 4
Cannabis, edited by David T. Brown

Volume 5
Neem, edited by H.S. Puri

Volume 6
Ergot, edited by Vladimír Křen and Ladislav Cvak

Volume 7
Caraway, edited by Éva Németh

Volume 8
Saffron, edited by Moshe Negbi

Volume 9
Tea Tree, edited by Ian Southwell and Robert Lowe

Volume 10
Basil, edited by Raimo Hiltunen and Yvonne Holm

Volume 11
Fenugreek, edited by Georgios Petropoulos

Volume 12
Gingko biloba, edited by Teris A. Van Beek

Volume 13
Black Pepper, edited by P.N. Ravindran

Volume 14
Sage, edited by Spiridon E. Kintzios

Volume 15
Ginseng, edited by W.E. Court

Volume 16
Mistletoe, edited by Arndt Büssing

Volume 17
Tea, edited by Yong-su Zhen

Volume 18
Artemisia, edited by Colin W. Wright

Volume 19
Stevia, edited by A. Douglas Kinghorn

Volume 20
Vetiveria, edited by Massimo Maffei

Volume 21
Narcissus and Daffodil, edited by Gordon R. Hanks

Volume 22
Eucalyptus, edited by John J.W. Coppen

Volume 23
Pueraria, edited by Wing Ming Keung

Volume 24
Thyme, edited by E. Stahl-Biskup and F. Sáez

Volume 25
Oregano, edited by Spiridon E. Kintzios

Volume 26
Citrus, edited by Giovanni Dugo and Angelo Di Giacomo

Volume 27
Geranium and Pelargonium, edited by Maria Lis-Balchin

Volume 28
Magnolia, edited by Satyajit D. Sarker and Yuji Maruyama

Volume 29
Lavender, edited by Maria Lis-Balchin

Volume 30
Cardamom, edited by P.N. Ravindran and K.J. Madhusoodanan

Volume 31
Hypericum, edited by Edzard Ernst

Volume 32
Taxus, edited by H. Itokawa and K.H. Lee

Volume 33
Capsicum, edited by Amit Krishna De

Volume 34
Flax, edited by Alister Muir and Niel Westcott

Volume 35
Aloe, edited by Tom Reynolds

Volume 36
Cinnamon and Cassia, edited by P.N. Ravindran, K. Nirmal Babu and M. Shylaja

Volume 37
Utrica, edited by Gulsel Kavalali

Volume 38
Kava, edited by Yadhu N. Singh

Kava

From ethnology to pharmacology

Edited by

Yadhu N. Singh

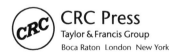

CRC Press
Taylor & Francis Group
Boca Raton London New York

CRC Press is an imprint of the
Taylor & Francis Group, an **informa** business

A TAYLOR & FRANCIS BOOK

First published 2004 by Taylor & Francis

Published 2019 by CRC Press
Taylor & Francis Group
6000 Broken Sound Parkway NW, Suite 300
Boca Raton, FL 33487-2742

© 2004 by Taylor & Francis Group, LLC
CRC Press is an imprint of Taylor & Francis Group, an Informa business

First issued in paperback 2019

No claim to original U.S. Government works

ISBN 13: 978-0-367-44659-8 (pbk)
ISBN 13: 978-0-415-32327-7 (hbk)

Visit the Taylor & Francis Web site at
http://www.taylorandfrancis.com

and the CRC Press Web site at
http://www.crcpress.com

Typeset in Garamond by
Integra Software Services Pvt. Ltd, Pondicherry, India

British Library Cataloguing in Publication Data
A catalogue record for this book is available from the British Library

Library of Congress Cataloging-in-Publication Data
Kava : from ethnology to pharmacology / edited by Yadhu N Singh
  p.   cm. — (Medicinal and aromatic plants—industrial profiles; v. 38)
  Includes bibliographical references and index.
  ISBN 0–415–32327–4 (hardback: alk. paper)
  1. Kava plant.   2. Kava plant—Therapeutic use.   3. Kava (Beverage)
  [DNLM: 1. Kava.   2. Plants, Medicinal.   3. Anti-Anxiety Agents—therapeutic use.
  4. Plant Extracts—therapeutic use. QV 766 K21 2003]   I. Singh,
  Y.N. (Yadhu Nand)   II. Series.

  RM666 .K38K38 2003
  615'.32325—dc21

                                                                2003008341

ISBN 0–415–32327–4

Original cover illustration by V. Lebot, reproduced with permission from the National Tropical Botanical Garden, Hawaii, USA.

Contents

List of contributors   vi
Preface   vii

1 An Introduction to Kava *Piper methysticum*   1
   YADHU N. SINGH

2 History, Folklore, Traditional and Current Uses of Kava   10
   LAMONT LINDSTROM

3 Kava: Production, Marketing and Quality Assurance   29
   YADHU N. SINGH

4 Botany and Ethnobotany of Kava   50
   YADHU N. SINGH

5 Chemistry of Kava and Kavalactones   76
   IQBAL RAMZAN AND VAN HOAN TRAN

6 Pharmacology and Toxicology of Kava and Kavalactones   104
   YADHU N. SINGH

7 Kava: Clinical Studies and Therapeutic Implications   140
   NIRBHAY N. SINGH, SUBHASHNI D. SINGH AND YADHU N. SINGH

Index   165

Contributors

Lamont Lindstrom
Department of Anthropology
University of Tulsa
Tulsa, OK 74104
USA

Iqbal Ramzan
Department of Pharmaceutics
Faculty of Pharmacy
The University of Sydney
Sydney, NSW 2006
Australia

Nirbhay N. Singh
ONE Research Institute
7401 Sparkleberry Lane
Chesterfield, VA 23832
USA

Subhashni D. Singh
ONE Research Institute
7401 Sparkleberry Lane
Chesterfield, VA 23832
USA

Yadhu N. Singh
Department of Pharmaceutical Sciences
College of Pharmacy
South Dakota State University
Box 2202C
Brookings, SD 57007
USA

Van Hoan Tran
Department of Pharmaceutics
Faculty of Pharmacy
The University of Sydney
Sydney, NSW 2006
Australia

Preface

In the past few decades, kava has become known throughout the world for its calming and relaxing properties. But before that, it was extensively used in the Pacific in most islands of Polynesia and Melanesia and significant parts of Micronesia, at least until the full impact of contact with Europeans in the form of colonization and missionization was felt by the inhabitants. Just as the potential therapeutic benefits of this herb in the treatment of stress, anxiety, insomnia, and restlessness began to be recognized, reports of its alleged involvement in cases of liver toxicity started appearing in the West. Consequently, the demand for commercial preparations of kava has been severely curtailed. However, its consumption in the traditional beverage form has continued unabated, both in the South Pacific and other parts of the world, as its use has never been associated with any organ dysfunction except for a scaly skin condition, called kava dermopathy, which appears in habitual consumers of excessive quantities of the drink.

In addition to organizations and individuals elsewhere, the governments and other institutions in the kava-producing countries are promoting initiatives in the form of scientific, medical, social, and economic research to elucidate the pharmacological and toxicological properties of this herb and to evaluate its full therapeutic and market potential. Hopefully the studies will also identify the origins of the kava-induced liver toxicity. These endeavors are of vital importance because of the serious impact the case reports have had not only on the economic viability of these small island nations but also to safeguard the health status of their citizens and others who continue to consume kava. Furthermore, kava represents an attractive alternative to some antistress and antianxiety agents which are known to have severe adverse effects. Thus, it is my sincere hope that this book will prove to be a valuable resource for these and other related activities by the interested parties as they proceed with their investigations to resolve this controversy.

In the preparation of this volume, I have been fortunate to receive the assistance and counsel of a number of people to whom I extend my heartfelt gratitude. In particular, I wish to thank the chapter authors, Drs Lamont Lindstrom, Iqbal Ramzan, Nirbhay Singh, Van Hoan Tran, and Ms Subhashni Singh. I also thank Mr Prakash Singh, Mr Yatesh Singh, Dr John Brown, Dr Pierre Cabalion, Dr Richard Davis, Mr Frank King, Ms Judy Siers, Dr Patricia Siméoni, and Dr Sadaquat Ali who all kindly provided materials for some of the illustrations.

Finally, I would like to dedicate this volume to the three people who matter most in my life, my wife Kamal, for all her love, encouragement, and support, and our children Yatesh and Kashmir.

Yadhu N. Singh

1 An Introduction to Kava *Piper methysticum*

Yadhu N. Singh

I can remember the evening gatherings when I was young at my home in the Fiji Islands when kava stock was pounded into powder in wooden mortars with metal rods, and then used in the preparation of the characteristic infusion. As I grew older it fell to me more and more often to purchase the kava from the neighborhood store, do the pounding and preparing of the beverage, and serve it to the assembled people, who invariably were men. It was only later when I was much older that I could appreciate the various facets of the process and the historical and cultural rationale and significance for them.

The kava buyer was told to always purchase the lateral roots and rootlets (called *waka* in Fiji) as the best drink was prepared from them. Next in preference were the thickened underground parts of the stem and stump comprising the rhizome (*lewena*). The *kasa* (the first few nodes and internodes of the stem or stalk) of the plant was acceptable only if the *waka* or *lewena* was unavailable. On no account was already powdered kava to be used, as it might have been derived from the stalks, or a mixture of stalks and root, and there was the possibility of adulteration with sawdust, flour, soil, or other contaminants. Furthermore, the drinkers often examined and smelled the rootstock for freshness as deterioration occurs with storage (Duve and Prasad, 1983). In addition to potency, the older material also loses its characteristic odor and flavor, both of which are highly relished by the drinkers.

Kava is an attractive shrub (Figure 1.1) that is propagated vegetatively, as are most of the traditional Pacific crops. The active principles are a group of psychoactive chemicals called kavalactones or kavapyrones (Chapter 5), which are concentrated mostly in the rhizome and roots, and in other parts of the plants to a lesser extent. The desired physiological effects are obtained by ingesting the active compounds present in cold-water infusions of ground, macerated, pounded, or sometimes chewed kava stumps and roots.

It has now been shown that those cultivars with high proportions of the kavalactone kavain (or kawain) give the more palatable drink and produce pleasant and desirable physiological effects. Cultivars that have high levels of dihydrokavain and dihydromethysticin are unpopular and, if possible, avoided by drinkers (Lebot and Brunton, 1985). Thus, although many cultivars have been available, the process of selection by kava users has reduced to a small number the cultivars that are most commonly propagated and utilized for recreational purposes.

The preparation of the beverage must be done in the proper manner to ensure that the strength of the drink is to the liking of the imbibers. A weak infusion is not well regarded, and could be the cause of major embarrassment to the host. The habit of

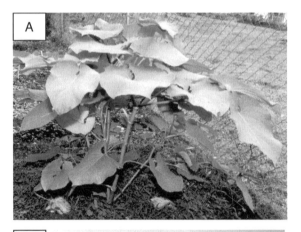

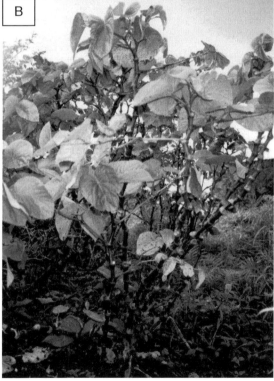

Figure 1.1 Kava plants of two different cultivars from the Fiji Islands. The plants are (A) six months and (B) two-years old. Note the differences in the color and structural characteristics of the leaves and stems. (B) Reprinted from Singh (1992), Kava, an overview, *Journal of Ethnopharmacology*, 37, 13–45, with permission from Elsevier Science.

pouring a little of the drink at the edge of the mat before consuming it is performed as a libation to the gods. The practice had become so ingrained in the kava custom that even people of non-Pacific origin like my father and his colleagues, most of who were descendants of Indian migrants, thought nothing of performing it on a regular basis.

Other aspects of the traditional practices that I remember include the drinking of the whole potion in one movement and the clapping of hands, usually three times, after each participant had finished his turn. As discussed in Chapter 2 and elsewhere (e.g., Singh, 1992), these are all integral parts of the kava ceremony, irrespective of the degree of its formality. Thus, the common use of kava in island communities, even among people of different cultural origins, maintains many of the practices that developed over centuries before the arrival of explorers, travelers, and missionaries. A typical kava social circle is depicted in Figure 1.2.

The term Oceania was applied by early European explorers to the island countries of the Pacific Ocean, in particular to the three cultural or ethnic groups of Polynesia, Melanesia, and Micronesia (Figure 1.3). The words are derived from the Greek words *melanos* (black pigment), *polys* (many), *mikros* (small), and *nesos* (island). The three cultural groupings are not mutually exclusive as there are many instances of intermingling of races and cultures. Archeological evidence indicates that human occupation of the Pacific islands began at least 20,000 years ago from South East Asia. While the settlement of Melanesia continued from 20,000 to 10,000 years ago, migrations to Micronesia and Polynesia began only some 3000–4000 years ago. The often held view that Pacific Islanders came in separate waves of "pure" races is refuted by evidence from the latest archaeological and blood-type genetic studies. These indicate a more complex process of mixing and differentiation which is also reflected in the systems of indigenous medicine and cultural practices (Siwatibau, 1997).

Oceania was, besides North America, the only cultural area which apparently did not have alcoholic beverages at the time of the first significant contact with Europeans in

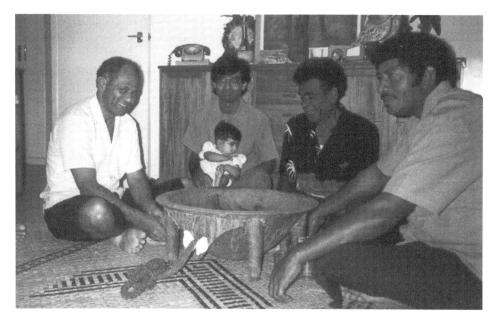

Figure 1.2 A kava drinking party in the Fiji Islands with the author (holding his four month old daughter) and his indigenous Fijian friends.

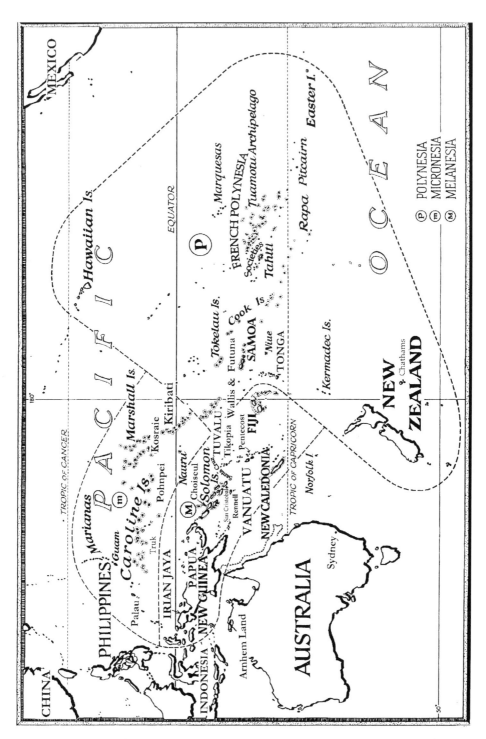

Figure 1.3 Map of the Pacific Ocean showing the three cultural regions of Melanesia, Micronesia and Polynesia. Modified from *Fiji in Colour* by Jim Siers, and reproduced with permission from the author.

the eighteenth century. However, many of the islands possessed the drink generally called kava. Like alcohol elsewhere, it had acquired for itself certain symbolic meanings and had associated with it a number of rules and procedures for its preparation, serving, and consumption.

The importance of kava in Oceania should perhaps be considered in the context that most cultures have their own psychoactive materials and, in spite of their great diversity, they have had the same kind of social status and significance (Serpenti, 1969). The sociological role of kava may be compared to that of peyote in many native or indigenous tribes of North America, coca leaves with communities in South America, and opium and related substances in the Middle and Far East. Previously, the kava custom was so widespread in Oceania that it may be considered to be the one item of their material culture that linked together most of the peoples of that part of the world (Singh, 1992).

Besides being the favored drink of chiefs and noblemen, it has also been used: to welcome distinguished visitors, such as visiting heads of states including royalty, presidents, prime ministers and the Pope (Singh and Blumenthal, 1997); at initiation and completion of work in the villages, like house or boat building (Turner, 1861; Mead, 1930); to cure illnesses and remove curses (Mariner, 1827); in preparing for a journey or an ocean voyage; installation in office (Gifford, 1929); in validation of titles; in ratification of agreements; in celebration of important births, marriages, and deaths (Mead, 1930); as a prelude to tribal wars (Newell, 1947); as a libation to the gods (Firth, 1970) – in fact, in virtually all aspects of life in the islands.

The English explorer, Captain James Cook, who visited the South Pacific in the eighteenth century, noted in his log that some members of his crew sampled large doses of kava and appeared to experience symptoms similar to those induced by opium (Cook, 1785). His botanical artist Daniel Scholander prepared in 1769 one of the first drawings of the plant that survives to the present day (Figure 1.4) and is deposited in the Natural History Museum in London. Although Cook's description is not completely accurate, as kava is neither hallucinogenic nor stupefying, it nevertheless alludes to the psychoactivity of the substance.

Kava has been difficult to categorize in modern scientific drug classification systems given its complex and subtle psychoactive properties. In large part, this is due to the presence in it of six major active components, the kavalactones, which exhibit pharmacological activity and are present in proportions which are dependent on various genetic and environmental factors.

A critical and objective appraisal of the effects of kava drinking indicates that kava produces relatively pleasant effects, especially in experienced drinkers, including feelings of sociability, peace, harmony, brotherhood, reduced anxiety and stress, muscle relaxation, and sedation. In higher doses, it may induce sleep. For instance, Hocart (1929) wrote that, "It gives a pleasant, warm and cheerful, but lazy feeling, sociable, though not hilarious or loquacious; the reason is not obscured," and Lemert (1967) observed, "...you feel friendly, not beer sentimental; you cannot fight with kava in you." However, there are other reports which speak unfavorably of this substance. Consider Torrey's (1848) report from the Marquesas:

Copious draughts cause a dizziness and a horribly distorted countenance. They lose the use of their limbs and fall and roll about on the ground, until the stupefication wears away.

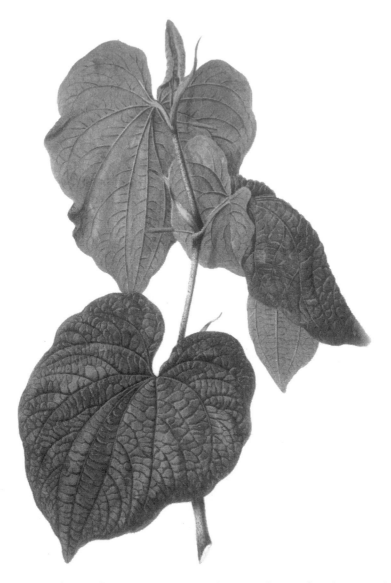

Figure 1.4 One of the earliest surviving drawings (from 1769) of *Piper methysticum* by Daniel Scholander. Note that the plant is denoted in the drawing as *P. inebrians*, re-named *P. methysticum* by Captain Cook's botanist Johann Forster. Reproduced with permission from the Natural History Museum, London.

Titcomb (1948) quotes a report by a Hawaiian, Kaualilinoe, written in the nineteenth century:

> There is no admiration for the body and face of an awa drinker whose eyes are sticky and whose skin cracks like the bark of the *kukui* trees of Lilikoi in unsightliness. If you are drunk with awa, you will find your muscles and cords limp, the head feels weighted and the whole body too.

As with many other substances, like alcohol, tobacco, and coffee, the kava beverage for most people has an acquired taste. Thus in naïve users, a number of adverse effects may be noted including headache and nausea, especially if a high dose is consumed. Authors who are unused to kava or are unsympathetic to it have described its taste and effects in fairly negative terms, comparing it to washing-up water, muddy water, "chalk swimming in body sweat," etc.

The etymology of kava is discussed in detail in Chapter 4 (section on *Traditional Classification and Etymology*). However, a brief introduction to the subject here will clarify the use of synonyms and their derivatives that may be encountered in earlier chapters. Although the term *kava* is the most recognized name, variants such as *kawa, kava-kava,* and *kawa-kawa* are often encountered. Furthermore, the initial *k* may be omitted, particularly in Polynesia, and they may become *ava, awa, ava-ava,* and *awa-awa,* or *'ava, 'awa, 'ava-ava,* and *'awa-awa.* In Fiji, a completely new word, *yaqona* (pronounced as *yangona* or *yanggona*) is used for kava. The names of the active kavalactones and other constituents (Figure 5.1) are derived from these terms, and the botanical name for kava, *P. methysticum.* Thus, the origin of methysticin obviously is from *methysticum,* yangonin from the Fijian term *yaqona,* kawain from kawa, and kavain from kava. Recently, the term kavain has started to supersede kawain in the scientific literature. Sometimes the former is used to indicate the racemic mixture resulting from chemical synthesis, that is (±)-kavain, and the latter for the naturally occurring compound which is a dextro-isomer, (+)-kawain. However, for all intents and purposes, the two terms, kavain and kawain, are beginning to be used interchangeably in the scientific literature.

Following the evolution of kava into a domesticated crop and food item, it became an integral commodity in the daily life of the island communities. But, with the impact of various outside influences relating to colonization, evangelical work by missionaries and conversion of the indigenous populations to Christianity, introduction of the more pharmacologically potent alcohol, and the slow disruption of the traditional way of life, the role of kava gradually declined in some places and virtually disappeared in others. However, in the last two to three decades of the twentieth century, there has been an upsurge of interest in the plant. There are distinct and different factors that probably were responsible, several of which are mentioned by Lebot *et al.* (1997). For linguists and prehistorians, its distribution together with those of other common Pacific crops provide clues to the migratory patterns of Oceanic peoples; for anthropologists and sociologists, it facilitates social interaction; botanists are fascinated by the problems of defining the species and by the sterility of its cultivars; for the theologically inclined, the practices relating to the kava offering and libations are of religious relevance; plant geneticists are surveying its chemotypes and zymotypes; villagers view the plant as a valuable cash crop much suited to traditional subsistence agriculture, while at the national level it could provide much needed export earnings for newly independent countries which are trying to build a sound economic base; and for the medical profession, which is interested in identifying from natural sources and traditional medical systems useful new therapies.

In the following chapters, various aspects of kava are discussed:

In Chapter 2, Dr Lamont Lindstrom addresses the history and folklore, including various myths and legends of the origin of kava from different countries; traditional and present uses of the plant and its products, including ceremonial, social, magico-religious, and medicinal; methods of preparation, including pounding and chewing to prepare the kavastock for making the infusion; the utensils used; and emerging use in the western healthcare systems.

Chapter 3, by Dr Yadhu Singh, describes the cultivation, diseases and pests, harvesting, drying and storage of kava; marketing and economic aspects, including kava as a cash crop, trading systems and networks that have been established locally, countrywide, and internationally for distribution to recreational users and the pharmaceutical and nutraceutical industry; quality assurance to safeguard against adulterants when used as a beverage, cultivar selection, recommended storage conditions, and procedures and standards used in industrial manufacturing.

The botany and ethnobotany of kava are discussed in Chapter 4 by Dr Yadhu Singh. The geographical distribution of the kava plant and the kava custom, both historical and current, are outlined, together with traditional classification of cultivars, etymology, and plant morphology. Taxonomy and nomenclature are also described. Chemotypic, zymotypic, and morphological data are discussed to clarify the botanic origins of kava by domestication of wild progenitors, and distribution pathways across the Pacific Ocean.

In Chapter 5, Dr Iqbal Ramzan and Dr Van Hoan Tran deal with the chemistry of the major psychoactive principles of kava, the kavalactones. The historical identification of the compounds, their molecular structures, distribution in plants, physico-chemical properties and pharmacokinetic behavior, structure–activity relationships, and identification of kava chemotypes are presented.

The pharmacology and toxicology of kava and kavalactones are summarized in Chapter 6 by Dr Yadhu Singh. He evaluates the early biological studies on kava extract, the pharmacodynamic actions of the extract and the pure components on anesthesia, sedation, local analgesia, local anesthesia, muscle function, and various effects originating in the central nervous system. The mechanisms which may account for the pharmacological actions are discussed with reference to the effects of kava extract and the kavalactones on ion channels, neurotransmitter release, GABAergic and benzodiazepine receptors, and monoamine uptake carriers. The chapter then considers the possible adverse effects which could occur with the use of kava and kava products. They include the effects on the skin, development of tolerance and dependence, interactions with foods, food supplements, and pharmaceutical drugs, mutagenicity, carcinogenicity, teratogenicity and the recently reported hepatotoxicity. In light of these possible toxic effects which may occur, precautions that need to be observed when using kava are outlined.

In Chapter 7, Dr Nirbhay Singh, Ms Subhashni Singh, and Dr Yadhu Singh discuss the clinical studies which have been done on the drug, and the therapeutic implications of these findings. They review the traditional roles of kava in healthcare and disease management, the data obtained from clinical studies on the efficacy of kava and kava preparations on anxiety syndrome, stress, restlessness, insomnia and quality of sleep, climacteric-related symptomatology, and cognitive function and information processing.

References

Cook, J. (1785) *A Voyage to the Pacific Ocean by the Command of his Majesty for Making Discoveries in the Southern Hemisphere*, Nicoll and Cadell, London, Vol. 1, pp. 318–319.

Duve, R.N. and Prasad, J. (1983) Changes in chemical composition of "yaqona" (*Piper methysticum*) with time. *Fiji Agriculture Journal*, 45, 45–50.

Firth, R. (1970) *Rank and Religion in Tikopia*, George Allen and Unwin, London, pp. 199–232.

Gifford, E.W. (1929) *Tongan Society*, Bulletin No. 61, Bernice P. Bishop Museum Press, Honolulu, pp. 156–170.

Hocart, A.M. (1929) *Lau Islands, Fiji*, Bulletin No. 62, Bernice P. Bishop Museum Press, Honolulu, pp. 59–70.

Lebot, V. and Brunton, R. (1985) *Tropical Plants as Cash Crops: A Survey of Kava in Vanuatu*, Vanuatu Department of Agriculture, Port Vila.

Lebot, V., Merlin, and Lindstrom, L. (1997) *Kava, the Pacific Elixir*, Healing Arts Press, Rochester, Vermont.

Lemert, E.M. (1967) Secular use of kava in Tonga. *Quarterly Journal of Studies on Alcohol*, **28**, 328–341.

Mariner, W. (1827) *An Account of the Natives of the Tonga Islands in the South Pacific Ocean*, John Martin, Edinburgh, Vol. 2, pp. 150–189.

Mead, M. (1930) *Social Organization of Manu'a*, Bulletin No. 76, Bernice P. Bishop Museum Press, Honolulu, pp. 102–112.

Newell, N.H. (1947) Kava ceremony in Tonga. *Journal of the Polynesian Society*, **56**, 364–417.

Serpenti, L.M. (1969) On the social significance of an intoxicant. *Tropical Man*, **2**, 31–44.

Singh, Y.N. (1992) Kava: an overview. *Journal of Ethnopharmacology*, **37**, 13–45.

Singh, Y.N. and Blumenthal, M. (1997) Kava: an overview. Distribution, mythology, botany, culture, chemistry, and pharmacology of the South Pacific's most revered herb. *HerbalGram*, **39**, 34–55.

Siwatibau, S. (1997) Medicine in the Pacific islands. In H. Selin (ed.), *Encyclopaedia of the History of Science, Technology, and Medicine in Non-Western Cultures*, Kluwer Academic Publishers, Dordrecht, pp. 709–714.

Titcomb, M. (1948) Kava in Hawaii. *Journal of the Polynesian Society*, **57**, 105–171.

Torrey, W. (1848) *Torrey's Narrative, or the Life and Adventures of William Torrey*, A.J. Wright, Boston, pp. 117–118.

Turner, G. (1861) *Nineteen Years in Polynesia*, J. Snow, London, pp. 122–123.

2 History, Folklore, Traditional and Current Uses of Kava

Lamont Lindstrom

Geographic Distribution of Kava and Kava Use

Kava's traditional distribution

Kava is a vegetatively propagated cultigen. Its presence in an environment, therefore, signals human cultivation and use of the plant. Along with tropical staples such as yam (*Dioscorea* spp.) and taro (*Colocasia* spp.; *Alocasia* spp.), kava grows throughout much of the tropical Pacific. Our knowledge of the traditional distribution of kava begins in the late eighteenth and early nineteenth centuries when sustained observation of Pacific Island cultures began. The exact boundaries of kava use have no doubt fluctuated since its domestication some 3000 years ago given the vicissitudes of Pacific environments, population movements, and also people's choices to either take up or abandon use of the plant. At the time of initial European observations, kava cultivation and consumption extended from Pohnpei to Hawai'i in the northern Pacific, and from Fiji to the Austral Islands in the southern Pacific. People planted and drank kava in parts of all three of the standard geographic regions into which the island Pacific is divided (Brunton, 1989; Lebot *et al.*, 1992; Singh, 1992). Most Polynesians, many Melanesians, and some Micronesians used the plant historically, and large numbers continue to do so today (Figure 2.1).

In Polynesia, kava existed in all the major high island groups (Samoa, Tonga, Cook Islands, Hawai'i, Wallis and Futuna, the Marquesas, and the Society Islands including Tahiti). It did not grow in New Zealand, where the climate is too cold for *Piper methysticum* or *P. wichmannii*, on Easter Island and Rapa, located on Polynesia's eastern fringe, or on the atolls and low-lying islets of Kiribati, Tuvalu, the Tuamotus, and the Chathams. In Melanesia, people throughout Fiji and Vanuatu (except perhaps for some mountainous areas of Malakula, Espiritu Santo, and Ambrym) cultivated and used kava. Kava was not planted in New Caledonia, the Loyalties, or the Solomon Islands, although a few historical reports have placed it in parts of San Cristobal, the Santa Cruz group, and also the Polynesian outliers Tikopia and Anuta (all part of today's Republic of the Solomon Islands). Kava is known in a few regions on the large island of New Guinea (which is divided into Papua New Guinea in the east and the Indonesian province of Irian Jaya or West Papua in the west) and also its neighboring archipelagos. These locales include the Admiralty Islands, the northeastern coastal areas of Madang and Morobe Provinces of Papua New Guinea, and the southern border regions of that country and West Papua. Finally, in Micronesia, at time of first contact, kava was found on only two of the Caroline Islands: Pohnpei and Kosrae.

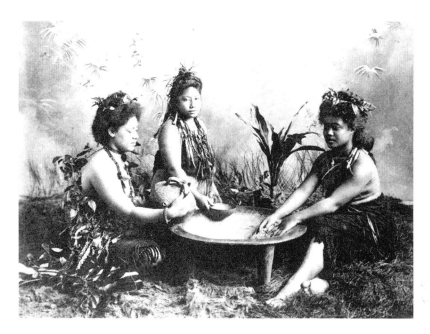

Figure 2.1 Kava making in Fiji in the early 1900s. From a postcard published by Robbie and Co. Ltd, Levuka, Fiji.

Contemporary kava distribution

After two centuries of colonialization and missionization, kava's distributive range has decreased. Regular cultivation and use of the drug today occur only in Vanuatu, Fiji, Samoa, Tonga, Wallis and Futuna, Pohnpei, and a few scattered regions of New Guinea. Recently, however, a number of Australian Aboriginal communities have taken up kava drinking, as have some urbanites in Noumea, New Caledonia. And, associated in part with political sovereignty movements and a growing market for kavalactones, the plant is undergoing something of a revival in Hawai'i and, to a lesser extent, French Polynesia (e.g., in Tahiti). A number of growers, particularly on the big island of Hawai'i, have expanded kava plantings. Endeavors are underway at the University of Hawai'i, the University of the South Pacific, and elsewhere to explore the plant's commercial possibilities within the Pacific and beyond.

By the mid-1990s, thousands of North Americans, Europeans, and Australians had begun using kava products as an alternative medicine and herbal relaxant. Drug stores and supermarkets offer a variety of kava products in pill, capsule, tea, and liquid form. In addition, powdered kava root is available by mail order from a number of websites (e.g., www.fijian-kava.com, www.shamansgarden.com, www.kickbackwithkava.com, www.fijilive.com, etc.). Most of this exported kava derives from Fiji and Vanuatu, and to a lesser extent, Samoa and Tonga.

Origin Myths

Numerous myths circulate in kava-using societies that account for the plant's origins and its powers. Despite this variety, it is possible to abstract common themes from these stories (see Lebot *et al.*, 1992). Important themes include associations of kava with both death and rebirth, and with masculinity versus femininity. Many myths trace kava's origins to a buried, female corpse. The plant grows from the womb, or vagina, of the buried woman. A myth from Pentecost Island, Vanuatu, for example, highlights these themes of death and rebirth:

> A very long time ago, orphan twins, a brother and sister, lived happily on Maewo [an island just north of Pentecost]. One night the boy, who loved his sister very much, had to protect her from a stranger who had asked to marry her but whom she had refused. In the struggle the frustrated suitor loosed an arrow that struck the girl and killed her. In despair, the boy brought his sister's body home, dug a grave, and buried her. After a week, before any weeds had grown over her tomb, there appeared a plant of unusual appearance which he had never seen. It had risen alone on the grave. The boy decided not to pull it up. A year passed and the sorrowful boy still had not been able to quell the suffering he felt at his sister's death. Often he went to mourn by her grave. One day he saw a rat gnaw at the plant's roots and die. His immediate impulse was to end his own life by eating large amounts of these roots, but when he tried, instead of dying, he forgot all his unhappiness. So he came back often to eat the magic root and taught its use to others.
>
> (Cited in Lebot *et al.*, 1992)

Origin myths such as this often serve as social "charters." People cite them to legitimate contemporary behavioral patterns and understandings. Kava myths, in this way, charter particular ritual and everyday uses of the drug. This Pentecost Island myth, for example, repeats widespread metaphoric understandings of kava intoxication as a sort of death – a death that precedes rebirth. Kava shoots from the woman's body. The plant both originates in death – growing from the woman's body – and causes death. But this second death (i.e., intoxication) likewise leads to a rebirth. The mournful brother, copying the rat, attempts to kill himself but instead discovers that kava has cured his grief. The myth combines two cycles of death and rebirth. In the first, the rejected suitor shoots an arrow into (inseminates) the girl and kills (impregnates her). From her buried corpse grows a kava plant (the child). Next, although this plant appears to cause death, intoxication in fact brings about a sort of new life as the brother overcomes his sorrow through kava.

Death is a common metaphorical understanding of drug-induced altered states of consciousness (Reichel-Dolmatoff, 1972; Turner, 1986). In some regions, people refer to kava as "poison," a term that reflects mythic interpretations of drunkenness as death. Drinkers on Tanna, Vanuatu, using the verb *akona* ("poison"), joke about how they "poison themselves with kava." In the Lau Islands of Eastern Fiji, "the intoxication caused by kava is called *mateni*, meaning death from or illness from. The expression *mate ni yanggona* [die from kava] is also used" (Hocart, 1929). People commonly induce altered states of consciousness in order to facilitate contact with ancestral and other spirits. Traditionally, they turned to these spirits for guidance and support. During the period in which they are "slain" or "poisoned" by kava, drinkers more easily engage the world of the dead.

Kava death is also a renewed life. Fijians, for example, sometimes refer to kava as "the water of life" (Turner, 1986). An origin myth from Samoa likewise celebrates kava's life-giving powers:

The deity Tagaloa Ui walked through a grove of kava plants and discovered the house of the mortal Pava. Pava invited the chief to enter his house and there the first kava ceremony involving mortal men was held...While Pava was wringing the kava, his son, Fa'alafi, laughed and played near the bowl. Tagaloa Ui instructed Pava to make the boy sit down and be quiet, but nothing was done about the irreverent boy. After several unheeded warnings, Tagaloa Ui picked up a coconut frond, formed it into a knife and cut Pava's son into two pieces. Then Tagaloa Ui said to Pava, "This is the food for the kava. This is your part and this is mine." Pava mourned and could not drink the kava...After preparing a second batch of kava from a special plant brought down from Tagaloa's mountain home, Tagaloa said, "Bring me my cup first." Tagaloa Ui did not drink this kava but poured it onto his piece of the dead son of Pava and then onto Pava's piece. Then he said, "*Soifua* (life)." The two parts came together and the boy lived.

(Holmes, 1961)

Understandings of kava as a life-giving fluid seemingly negate darker metaphors of kava as poison. The apparent contradiction here dissolves within broader cultural equations of birth and death within many Pacific cultures. Birth and death both are moments of passage from the world of the spirits to that of the living, or vice versa. Kava lubricates these transitions between two domains of existence. It moves living drinkers closer to spiritual realms so that they can better hear the voices of ancestors. It also enhances fertility and the eruption of new life – the materialization of the spiritual.

Some kava origin myths sexualize the plant itself. A myth from southeast Tanna takes note of kava's original phallic qualities:

Long ago when the ancestors were alive, two women gathered wild yams and went to scrape their peels off in a tide pool at the sea. Mwatiktiki [a hero associated with the neighboring island of West Futuna, and an avatar of Polynesia's Maui] had brought to Tanna a kava plant and had hidden it in a hole in rocks on shore. The two women squatted down and began to peel their yams. A kava shoot rose up and out, stuck into the vagina of one of the women, and began to do it. She said to herself, "I feel something good, something sweet!" The kava continued to do it. She turned to her sister and asked, "What is poking me?" They saw that it was kava. They pulled out the kava shoot and carried it back to their garden at Isouragi, where they planted it. At that time, men drank only wild kava. They had yet no knowledge of the real thing. The women weeded the kava plant in secret. They then dug it up, prepared food, and brought it to the kava-drinking ground and told men there that if they drank this kava they would feel something different. Men quit drinking wild kava and began using real kava. From that drinking ground, kava reached every area of the island.

(Lindstrom, 1987)

Kava root, in this myth, is a symbolic phallus. Its juices, along these lines, symbolically are a fertilizing fluid, either semen or breast milk. Fijians and Tongans call the struts on their kava bowls "breasts" rather than legs – breasts that offer up the life-giving drink (Figure 1.2). Kava's fertile properties account for its use in many Pacific folk medical and magical systems. On Malakula, for example, gardeners once poured libations of kava onto ancestral skulls to ensure bountiful yam harvests. The Marind-Anim of West Papua similarly conferred vital qualities on new canoes with kava libations (Baal, 1966).

If phallic kava fertilizes, then intoxication can be taken to be a sort of sexual experience. The sexualization of drug-induced states of consciousness is common in many cultures (Furst, 1972; Reichel-Dolmatoff, 1972). Male drunkenness, as a symbolically fertile state is, however, endangered by real sexual contact with women. This is the reason why the virgin boy or girl is the most appreciated kava maker in many island societies. The clean touch of these sexually uninitiated youngsters does not undermine or prevent men's kava intoxication. On Tanna, once a youth has sex he can no longer mix his elders' kava with his hands. In Samoa and Tonga, cere-monial village virgins (*taupou* or *tou'a*) prepare kava at important ritual occasions. In Vanuatu, people fear that recent sexual intercourse can prevent drinkers from feeling their kava. Conversely, indulgence in kava drinking also causes men to lose interest in sexual relations, as a Kiwai origin myth from southwestern Papua New Guinea asserts:

> The first *gamoda* [kava] sprang up at Sareeve from the dung of a kangaroo and was found by a Masingle man named Bege. During the night the plant came to him in a dream and taught him how to grow and drink it. He showed the people the use of it...From that time onward everybody planted gamoda in his garden. Bege said, "That gamoda belong man; no good woman he drink milk belong gamoda. Man he want *kobori* (have connection with) woman, he no drink him gamoda first, he no want gamoda go along woman" ["Gamoda belongs to men; it is not proper for women to drink the milk of the gamoda. Men who want intercourse with women should not first drink gamoda, they should not mix gamoda with women"].
> (Landtman, 1927)

Pacific Islanders recite their kava origin myths to account for common beliefs about the essential characteristics of the drug and for the rules that regulate its use. Notably, origin myths legitimate inequality of access to the drug. For example, throughout most of Melanesia only men had rights to drink kava. Although women, originally, may have discovered kava, as in the myth from Tanna above, they then misused it or were otherwise incapable of consuming the drug properly. Because of mythic female short-comings, or because of kava's presumed effects on women and their fertility, men reserved kava for themselves.

Only high ranking women within Polynesian and Micronesian chiefdoms such as Tonga, Samoa, Tahiti, and Pohnpei, and women elsewhere past menopause whose gender status typically becomes masculinized as they age, enjoyed kava drinking rights (Brunton, 1989). Kava is an important token of exchange and an avenue to supenatural inspiration. Women's chances to participate in political and religious arenas are diminished insofar as they have fewer rights to drink kava.

Botanic Origins

Kava origin myths sort into two types. The first recounts local origins of kava – its indigenous generation. Kava appears locally, often growing from a buried human corpse, typically out of the vagina of a woman. Humans observe an intoxicated rat, or sometimes a mouse or pig, that has dug up and chewed kava root and they thereby learn how to use kava – sometimes in conjunction with sugarcane, the sweetness of the latter overcoming the bitterness of the drug. The second type of origin myth tells of kava's external origins. Some god or cultural hero introduces the drug, importing kava from an overseas or spiritual locale (Lebot *et al.*, 1992).

Myths citing internal origins are one possible indicator of where people first domesticated *P. methysticum* (although mythic elements may diffuse even more easily than kava stem cuttings, and islanders who borrowed kava cuttings from abroad may also have borrowed foreign origin myths). Myths of internal kava origins occur in northern Vanuatu, Tonga, southern New Guinea, and Tikopia. Botanical evidence indicates that the first of these areas – northern Vanuatu – is kava's most likely point of origin (see Chapter 4). Kava subsequently diffused, along with certain myth motifs, to central Micronesia, coastal New Guinea, Fiji, and nuclear Polynesia (Samoa and Tonga) to then spread farther east to Hawai'i, Tahiti, and the Marquesas (where kava myths typically recount the plant's external origins).

Gaps in kava's distribution complicate theories of where the plant was first domesticated. Although used throughout most of Vanuatu, it was unknown in the Solomon Islands to the west. But still farther west, across the Solomons, kava occurred in sporadic locations on the main and offshore islands of New Guinea and, to the north, on two of the Caroline Islands. East of Vanuatu, people drank kava on most Polynesian islands that could support the plant. But just to the south, kava was again unknown in the Loyalty Islands and in New Caledonia. Contemplating these gaps, Brunton (1989) speculated that kava has been an "abandoned narcotic." First domesticated, perhaps, in the Bismarck Archipelago north of New Guinea, kava then spread eastward, possibly carried by ancestral Polynesian voyagers that archeologists have associated with Lapita-style pottery. Subsequently, if Brunton is correct, people in the Solomon Islands, the Santa Cruz, and Bismarck archipelagos gave up use of the drug, perhaps in the grip of some religious enthusiasm.

Vincent Lebot instead has argued that kava was first domesticated in northern Vanuatu, perhaps on Pentecost or Maewo Island (Lebot, 1989; Lebot and Lévesque, 1989). If he is correct, kava may never have diffused into the Solomon Islands where people already used betel, a second traditional drug substance comprising a mixture of areca palm kernel, lime, and the leaves, stems or catkins of another plant of the pepper family, *P. betle*. If kava did indeed originate in northern Vanuatu, it could have been carried northward to Pohnpei and Kosrae in Micronesia and, from there, southwestward to the coastal areas and islands off northern Papua New Guinea. Presumably, it might also have diffused directly from Vanuatu to southern coastal areas of New Guinea, bypassing the Solomon Islands, although distances here are great. Its transmission eastward would have been easier, given evidence of planned and unplanned prehistoric sea voyages between Vanuatu, Fiji, and central Polynesia. From Fiji as well as Tonga and Samoa, voyagers next carried the plant to the Cook Islands, Tahiti, the Marquesas, and Hawai'i. Nuclear Polynesian voyagers may also have brought kava back westward into southern Vanuatu, given similarities in kava preparation style and nomenclature in the two areas (Brunton, 1989; Lebot *et al.*, 1992; but see Siméoni, 2002).

Several sorts of evidence suggest that people first domesticated kava in northern Vanuatu. First, kava's wild progenitor – *P. wichmannii* – grows in Vanuatu and is still occasionally cultivated for medicinal purposes. Second, there is a greater diversity of *P. methysticum* morphotypes, chemotypes, and zymotypes in this archipelago than anywhere else in the Pacific. The complete set of five *P. methysticum* chemotypes, for example, occurs only in Vanuatu (Lebot *et al.*, 1992). Morphologically, the plant also is most diverse in this archipelago with around 80 locally recognized and named cultivars.

If Islanders began cultivating and cloning *P. wichmannii* ("wild kava" in Bislama, Vanuatu's Pidgin English) soon after they first settled the archipelago, then domesticated kava today results from 3000 or more years of farmer selection.

Kava and Society

Like many other psychoactive substances, kava is a social drug. Islanders drink kava together, in groups. Traditional understandings of the drug's effects underscore its sociability. Most Islanders believe that kava promotes peace and tranquility. Kava also requires time and effort to prepare, and preparation, too, is a social occasion. The plant has significant economic, political, religious, and medical functions, although the details of these differ from society to society. In areas where people use kava daily (Vanuatu, Fiji, Samoa, Tonga, Pohnpei, and Wallis and Futuna), the plant is of major importance within both the traditional and cash economies. Kava is a preeminent gift within ritual exchange systems. It is also, increasingly, a valuable cash crop. Kava serves certain medical and religious functions, although these are somewhat muted in today's mostly Christian Pacific. Islanders use kava to welcome guests, to mark the beginning and completion of work projects, prepare for journeys or voyages, install chiefs and validate titles, ratify agreements, celebrate births, marriages and deaths, mark the beginnings of warfare or feud, honor the spirits, and cure the sick (Singh, 1992).

Gifts of kava

Exchanges of kava lubricate social relationships. In fact, because of shared assumptions that kava intoxication promotes sociability, the plant is a particularly appropriate gift. In Fiji, if a son upsets his father, he can repair relations with a presentation of kava (Arno, 1992). Kinfolk and neighbors share roots from each other's plantations, a different person contributing kava to the kava circle or informal drinking club each time it meets. "A person who comes to drink *yaqona* with others brings some *yaqona* as his *sevusevu*, a mark of respect for the group. Even a very small amount constitutes the *sevusevu*, although as a practical matter a certain amount will be needed to keep the supply going during the evening" (Arno, 1992). Elsewhere, the communal consumption of kava strengthens a variety of local groups, such as work groups on Kolepom Island (West Papua).

More formally, people exchange gifts of kava on important occasions, particularly during rites of passage such as circumcisions, marriages, and funerals (Figure 2.2). On Tonga, the families of brides and grooms drink kava together to celebrate their new affinity. Years later, when either wife or husband passes away, these families again exchange kava roots to mark the dissolution of the marriage. In Fiji and also Pohnpei, kava exchange marks a man's acquisition of a chiefly title. When a Pohnpei high chief bestows a title on another, "he takes a cup of kava in both hands and raises it high before him, and says loudly, 'This is the coconut shell vessel of [such and such title]'." The new chief then drinks (Riesenberg, 1968).

As a valued gift, Islanders may dress up or wrap their kava presentations. On Pohnpei, families giving away large kava plants carry these to the community house while singing and blowing shell trumpets. "The kava bushes are frequently decorated with ornamental plants. Large bushes carried on a litter may have a stalk of croton or breadfruit inserted in them" (Riesenberg, 1968). On Tanna, similarly, people decorate the kava plants they

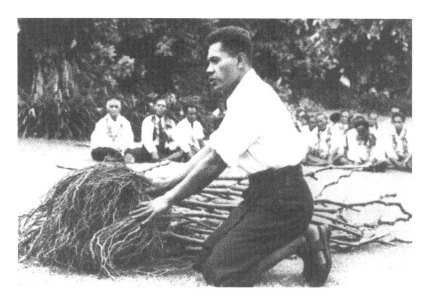

Figure 2.2 Ceremonial presentation of a large kava root with stems attached. Photo supplied by the Fiji Ministry of Information.

exchange at feasts celebrating the circumcision of their sons (Singh and Blumenthal, 1997). They strip the leaves from the branches and attach instead more colorful croton and cordyline leaves (Brunton, 1989). The circumcised boy's maternal uncle receives and drinks this festive kava in return for the care he provided the boy while his wound healed.

Kava exchange, in particular, celebrates the end of conflict and the achievement of good relations between families or villages – a peacemaking function that plays off people's perceptions that intoxication ensures tranquility and peacefulness, both within the person and within society. In Vanuatu, disputing parties who successfully resolve some conflict almost always exchange roots of kava, and often pigs and garden produce as well, to celebrate renewed good relations. They then drink kava together, both parties sharing kava for the first time since that conflict began. Similarly, in southwestern Papua New Guinea, part of a peace-making ceremony once consisted of men drinking kava: "During the drinking-feast one man of each side will sprinkle a little *gamoda* [kava] over the assembled people and say, 'No more fight now, no good you me [we] fight'" (Haddon, 1916).

Shared kava celebrates the restoration and maintenance of harmonious relations, but such relationships are not always egalitarian. In the chiefdoms of central and eastern Polynesia, and also Pohnpei, kava-drinking protocol demonstrates status difference. Various ceremonial procedures choreograph the chiefly kava circles of Samoa, Tonga, and Fiji, governing where people sit, the placement of the kava bowl, methods of preparation and service, and also drinking order. Kava circles remain an important political ritual today in Tonga, Samoa, and Fiji. In 1993, when King Taufa'ahau Tupou IV of Tonga visited Brigham Young University, Hawai'i campus, he convened a royal kava circle to bestow a chiefly title on the University's president.

Islanders have also adapted kava circles to contemporary needs. Churches and other community associations on Tonga, and also in Tongan immigrant communities in Hawai'i, California, and the cities of New Zealand and Australia, have transformed kava circles into money raising devices. In Honolulu, for example, Tongans gather weekly at Kapiolani and other seaside parks to drink kava. Participants in these kava circles place dollar bills on the head and shoulders of *tou'a* – the female kava preparers who also dance in the center of the circle. Kava circle organizers collect the money raised during the evening to support church or organizational needs.

Some uses of contemporary kava circles are what anthropologists call "rotating credit associations." Each week, a different participant takes home the proceeds of the evening – a sum of money he can use to cover extraordinary needs, such as airfare back to Tonga or a down payment on an automobile. Church-sponsored kava circles made the news in 2000 after several Tongans living in northern California were arrested on their way home for driving while intoxicated. The court, however, unsure whether kava ought to be equated with alcohol, exonerated two of the accused (Linden, 2000).

Like the Polynesian kava circle, Melanesians in Vanuatu have also updated and put to new uses their traditional *nakamal*, or men's house, where kava traditionally was prepared and consumed. Nowadays, scores of kava bars (also called *nakamal*) dot Vanuatu's capital, Port Vila (Figure 2.3). Kava is also on sale at Fijian marketplaces and in Noumea, New Caledonia (and there is at least one club that sells kava in Honolulu). Vanuatu's urban *nakamals* attract numerous drinkers each evening. A good proportion

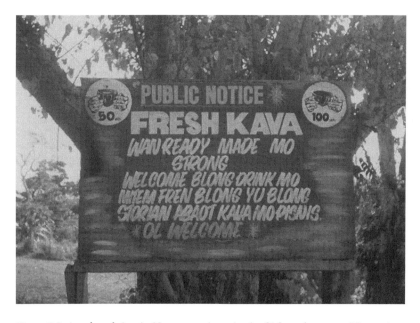

Figure 2.3 A *nakamal* sign in Vanuatu written in the Bislama language. The notice may be loosely translated as, "Fresh kava already prepared and strong. You are welcome to come and drink with your friends, to discuss kava and business. All welcome!" The sign also indicates that cups of kava cost 50 or 100 vatu. Photo by Lamont Lindstrom.

of Port Vila's businessmen, politicians, and civil servants choose kava over alcohol partly because of the plant's traditional resonance and partly because it is less expensive. The emergence of urban kava bars, beginning in the late 1970s, raised the commercial significance of Vanuatu kava as a cash crop (Lamboll, 1989; Kilham, 1996). This economic significance has increased further as kava markets have developed beyond the Pacific.

Kava has acquired new political functions as well as economic. Fiji, Vanuatu, Samoa, and the Federated States of Micronesia (including Pohnpei) achieved independence over the past four decades and have featured kava within evolving discourses of nationhood. Kava – the "traditional drink" – helps symbolize shared national identity. Samoa's two-*tala* (dollar) bill features a traditional wooden kava bowl (Figure 2.4). Kava drinking cups appear on Pohnpei's state flag and seal. Vanuatu has issued a postage stamp that celebrates "kava, the national plant," as has Wallis and Futuna depicting the whole plant (Figure 2.5). These symbolic uses of kava remind people of their larger political affiliations beyond the village – national unity here leans on kava's traditional solidarities.

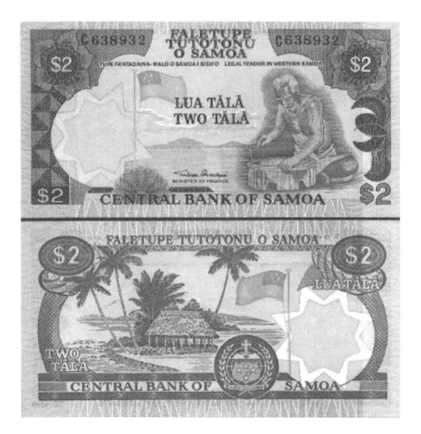

Figure 2.4 Samoa's two-*tala* (dollar) bill which on the obverse side features a man preparing kava in a traditional kava bowl (above). The reverse side shows a *fale*, a thatched hut without walls, where village meetings and often kava ceremonies are held (below).

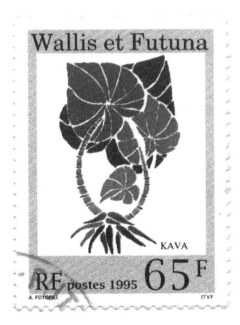

Figure 2.5 A postage stamp from Wallis and Futuna depicting a kava plant. Photo supplied by Pierre Cabalion.

Sacrifices of kava

If kava today links the drinker and the nation, traditionally, it connected humans with their gods and ancestral spirits. Most folk drugs that alter consciousness have significant religious uses (Schultes and Hofmann, 1979; Wasson, 1980). People understand intoxication or inebriation, as they also do dreams and trance, to be roads into the realm of the supernatural. Kava conjoins spirits and humans in two ways. First, people offer symbolic gifts of kava to gods and ancestors (Thompson, 1940; Titcomb, 1948; Riesenberg, 1968; Oliver, 1974). These sorts of kava sacrifices – gifts to the gods – parallel Islanders' everyday political exchange of kava among themselves. Second, kava induces an altered state of consciousness – delicate though this often is – that many drinkers claim facilitates their communication with the spirit world.

Men's enjoyment of kava in life presumably continues after death. The living, therefore, offer the dead symbolic gifts of kava, typically in the form of libations. For example, priests on Tikopia, a Polynesian outlier in the far eastern fringe of the Solomon Islands, sacrificed kava when asking for spiritual beneficence:

> First was an announcement to the god or ancestor invoked that the kava being performed was his, coupled with the citation of his personal name or title. This was to be construed as a personal association of the god with the rite, to secure his involvement … This was followed by a series of requests, according to circumstances, for growth of the crops, good harvest, a plentiful supply of fish at sea, calm weather, health for the people.
>
> (Firth, 1970)

Similar practices of pouring kava onto the ground for spiritual consumption occurs (or occurred) in Fiji (Roth, 1953; Toren, 1999), Tonga (Gifford, 1929; Newell, 1947); East Futuna (Burrows, 1936), West Futuna (Capell, 1960), Samoa (Churchill, 1916; Mead, 1930; Williamson, 1939; Holmes, 1961), northern Vanuatu (Rivers, 1914), and parts of New Guinea (Landtman, 1927).

Drinkers may also spit out a mouthful of kava, often the last in the cup. This, too, functions as a libation. On Tanna, men tip back large coconut shell cups of kava and, reaching the bottom of the cup, spit their last mouthful into the air. They then utter a short prayer or request to surrounding ancestors. These appeals – as on Tikopia – may be for good weather, for newly planted crops to grow, for health, for peace, or for one political party to win an upcoming election (Lindstrom, 1980). Kava spitting also occurs on Vanua Lava (Banks Islands): "after drinking the breath is blown out strongly (*pupsag*) in such a way that some of the kava is blown out too" (Rivers, 1914); and in Fiji: "a chief or a distinguished guest, after he has drunk his cup of *yanggona*, blows a small quantity of it through the lips against the wall of the house or away from his neighbors and then utters the name of some desired object or sentiment" (Roth, 1953). This spitting – the transmission of vital fluids from an inner to an outer domain – signifies the transmission of prayer, and kava, from one world to another.

In addition to facilitating the transmission of prayers and messages from humans to the spirits, kava also makes possible their reception. Drunk on kava, a man can overhear ancestral voices and thus tap into valuable knowledge. Kava is "universally recognized in the Pacific as a channel for divine (ancestral) inspiration" (Layard, 1942). Kava's power to alter consciousness is particularly important, given Pacific epistemology. Islanders value inspiration over creativity when explaining novel ideas. Knowledge passed down from ancestors, in one way or another, is worth more than an idea that an individual makes up on his own. Songwriters in Vanuatu, for example, seclude themselves and drink kava in order to overhear the spirits singing fragments of songs that they can later teach to others. They present these songs as ancestral communiqués rather than as the result of their own creative imaginations. Important men are buried on or near *nakamals* where men gather daily to prepare and drink kava. Ancestors, thus, literally surround kava drinkers and the drug prepares them to hear what the dead might be saying.

Folk metaphors of kava as a sort of poison, and of intoxication as a sort of death, play with the plant's powers to unite the living and the dead. In Fiji, for example, drunks claim to "die from kava" (Hocart, 1929). Kava's powers to link drinkers with the spirits are also apparent in the plant's divinational uses. Spirit mediums in Vanuatu may drink kava before divining the cause of someone's illness. In traditional Hawai'i, priests (*kahuna*) once diagnosed illness or discovered hidden information, such as the sex of unborn babies, by inspecting the movement of bubbles in cups of kava (Titcomb, 1948). Here again, kava served as a portal through which spiritual knowledge and advice flowed.

Most Islanders today are Christian (or Hindu or Muslim, in the case of Indo-Fijians) and kava's traditional religious uses have retreated. Many Christian missionaries, in fact, attempted for years to persuade their congregations not to drink kava – this is an understandable interdiction, given the plant's ability to link people with ancestral ghosts and gods. The church convinced people on Kosrae in the Caroline Islands and elsewhere to renounce kava. Mission hostility to kava was less prominent in Fiji and central Polynesia. Kava-drinking, here, remained associated with the political display of chiefly hierarchy, and these chiefs were commonly church leaders as well. As such, missionaries working in these societies overlooked kava's remnant pagan religious associations.

Attempts to prohibit kava-drinking waned after the Pacific War, particularly as new political ideologies emerged that celebrated kava as the "national drink" in newly independent states. Today, only a few Christian denominations such as the Seventh-Day Adventists and more fundamentalist newcomers such as the Holiness Fellowship or the Apostolic Church continue to attempt to prohibit kava drinking among their congregants. Some Christian denominations, in fact, building on kava's traditional spiritual associations, have incorporated use of the plant into their liturgies. Roman Catholics in Pohnpei, who were always less hostile to kava than were some of their Protestant compeers, employ kava in church rituals of atonement. Where islanders once presented kava to wronged chiefs in order to beg forgiveness, they now bring the plant to church, confess their sins, and request forgiveness from God. Priests, representing the deity, consume the drug as part of this atonement ceremony (McGrath, 1973). In Tonga, too, people present kava to church dignitaries during Sunday services, and also convene kava circles to welcome visiting preachers (Cowling, 1988). Pacific Islanders continue to offer up sacrifices of kava, although these gifts now are offered up to God alongside local ancestors and spirits. Kava carries one's prayers up to the supernatural; it also serves as a medium through which important inspirational knowledge and advice is received.

Doses of kava

Folk healers prescribe kava everywhere the drink is consumed. Island pharmacists gather various parts of the plant, including the root, leaves, bark, stems, and their juices. Treatments include infusions and also poultices of leaf, stem, or root applied to the body. Observers have recorded uses of kava to treat a range of conditions. These include urogenital and menstrual problems, headaches and migraines, asthma and other respiratory problems, toothache, boils, sores and wounds, conjunctivitis, both diarrhea and constipation, earache, sore throat, sleeping difficulties, leprosy and other skin diseases, and more (Lebot *et al.*, 1992; Kilham, 1996). Kava, occasionally, served also as an abortifacient (Riesenberg, 1968).

Some folk treatments have undoubted scientific validity given the plant's bactericidal, analgesic, diuretic, soporific, muscle relaxing, and calming properties. Other treatments may reflect kava's symbolic attributes. Use of the plant to induce milk flow in women, for example (Steinmetz, 1960), perhaps recalls the general appreciation of kava as a fertilizing fluid. Kava products were also introduced by European and American pharmaceutical manufacturers in the 1920s (Schübel, 1924) to treat insomnia, hypertension, and urogenital irritations.

In the 1990s, kava emerged as a popular item within the homeopathic and, more generally, the holistic health and herbal marketplace. Today, kavalactones, sometimes combined with other substances in tonics or capsules, are on sale as dietary supplements in health food stores, pharmacies, and supermarkets around the world. By 1998, kava sales in the US reportedly had grown to about $20 million. Kava is packaged and marketed principally as a treatment for anxiety and stress, although other benefits of the plant are also touted. Aloha Seed & Herb, for example, markets "Kava-for-Health" on the Internet:

Kava is best known as a relaxant, but it has a number of beneficial healing properties with no adverse side effects. Kava can be very effective at relieving depression and anxiety, improving mental ability, relaxing muscles, reducing pain, and lifting the mood by promoting feelings of well being and friendship. Kava also promotes deep, refreshing sleep with no grogginess after waking. Women find kava especially helpful for its ability to balance the hormones.

(www.kava-for-health.com, n.d.)

This source also sells kava candy, with "a soft center made from a 55% Vanuatu kava extract and sweetened with Fijian cane sugar. Excellent for a quick calm-down or even a scratchy throat."

Other manufacturers package extracts of kava for the recreational market. The brochure that accompanies small bottles of Black Fire ("Share the Experience! Kava-kava, Herbal Beverage") explains: "Works in seconds...Black Fire is pleasurable anytime, especially at the end of a busy day" (Hammer Corporation, n.d.). Kava concoctions are also occasionally on sale at adult bookstores, packaged as an aphrodisiac (and somewhat surprisingly so, given the anaphrodisiacal reputation that the drug has throughout most of the Pacific). Some Western consumers, suspicious that the kava extracts sold by the dietary supplement industry are weak, now buy powdered kava root from local retailers or on the Internet and infuse their own doses of the drug for health or recreational purposes.

Methods of Kava Preparation and Consumption

Techniques of kava preparation do more than just ready the plant material for consumption. Often, they are ritualized and elaborated to carry various sorts of religious and social meaning. Where supply permits, kava preparation is a daily ritual. Infused kava is never stored for the next day. Drinkers quickly polish off all that they prepare. In places where kava plantations are abundant and proximate, consumers typically prefer to drink kava "green." (Newly harvested kava no doubt offers higher concentrations of psychoactive kavalactones). Men dig up a plant in their plantation, or buy recently harvested kava roots in local markets, and prepare and drink this kava that day. Green rootstock, however, is not always immediately available and, in some societies, people have learned to preserve kava for future use by drying and then powdering the rootstock. In Vanuatu, New Guinea, Pohnpei, and Wallis and Futuna kava is consumed green, soon after it is harvested. In Fiji, Samoa, and Tonga the root is usually dried, sometimes powdered, and marketed for consumption elsewhere although people here, too, will sometimes drink green kava when available.

Kavalactones are more concentrated in the plant's roots rather than in its upper stems or leaves. Farmers thus carefully dig plants, root by root, taking care not to break the longer laterals that have a high percentage of kavalactones. Since kava is vegetatively propagated, harvesters cut away a plant's stems and cover these with soil. If that plant's effects on the body are appreciated, growers will return in several weeks and unearth its branches from the nodes of which new roots already will have sprouted for replanting.

If kava is to be dried for later consumption, growers wash the roots and then dry these either in the sun or in hot-air dryers (also used to produce copra, or dried coconut meat). After drying, producers pound or grind roots into a fine powder to be bagged and marketed. In places where people drink green kava, they use several techniques to macerate the rootstock and thus allow its kavalactones to infuse more readily in cold water. Maceration methods include masticating, grating, grinding, and pounding kava roots (which typically comprise a central woody rootstock surrounded by long lateral and shorter tertiary root – see Chapter 4).

Today, mastication of fresh kava occurs only in southern and parts of central Vanuatu, and in scattered locales in New Guinea. At one time, however, this method of preparation was common throughout Polynesia and Fiji (Beaglehole and Beaglehole, 1941; Titcomb, 1948). Men first broke up rootstock by pounding this into smaller pieces on a stone. Young virgin girls (or sometimes young boys, as is the case today in southern Vanuatu) were then obliged to masticate these pieces or the root. They eventually deposited mouthfuls of chewed pulp into large wooden bowls (*tanoa*) and then mixed and infused this pulp in cold water. They removed masticated residue, strained the drink, and then served this in half coconut shells to assembled drinkers (Steinmetz, 1960).

Polynesian and contemporary Fijian kava utensils include round wooden kava bowls supported on four or more legs (or "breasts" in local terms); cups carved from half coconut shells; and filters made from the inner bark of the hibiscus tree (*Hibiscus tiliaceus* – called *fau* in Samoa, *vau* in Fiji, and *'au* elsewhere). Hawaiian kava preparers also once used filters made from sedge fiber. Important kava bowls can measure up to several feet in diameter (Singh, 1992). Samoan, Tongan, and Fijian artisans today also produce these bowls for the tourist market, carved sometimes in the shape of turtles. Some modern Samoan bowls rest on numerous feet, sometimes as many as 30 (Figure 2.6). Fijian bowls may feature a sennit (coconut fiber) cord decorated with white cowrie shells that hangs from a lug carved into the bowl (Figure 1.2) and, when the bowl is in use, points towards the highest chief or most honored person sitting within the kava circle.

Kava chewing, as a mode of preparation, may have originated in Polynesia and subsequently diffused, from Tongan sources, to Fiji (along with kava bowls, coconut shell cups, and kava circles) and perhaps also southern Vanuatu. Fijians had adopted Tongan kava preparation and consumption practices by the mid-eighteenth century

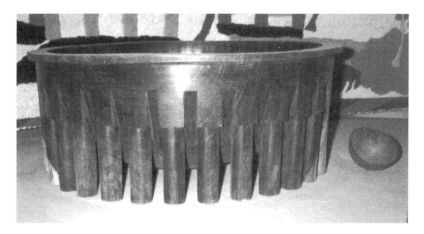

Figure 2.6 A multi (26)-legged tanoa from Samoa on display at the Samoan pavilion during *Expo* '86 in Vancouver, BC, Canada. A coconut shell cup lies next to the bowl. Photo by Yadhu Singh.

(Clunie, 1986). Previously, they had prepared rootstock by grinding and then infusing root grounds in shallow wooden bowls (of animal or human shape), in clay pots, or sometimes in leaf-lined holes dug into the ground. Drinkers sipped kava directly from these containers, sometimes using a straw, instead of making use of coconut shell cups as they do today. A century later, however, European missionaries and colonial administrators encouraged, or ordered, Fijians and Polynesians to abandon mastication as a matter of public hygiene. Islanders turned instead to grinding and pounding to process rootstock although chewing survived in some areas, such as East Futuna, until well into the twentieth century (Gaillot, 1962).

Mastication remains the main mode of processing kava root in southern and parts of central Vanuatu as well as in scattered locales in New Guinea (Knauft, 1987). On Tanna, for example, men first cut a freshly harvested kava root into a number of smaller pieces that they brush clean with coconut husks. Assisted by circumcised boys, they masticate a mouthful of kava root for fifteen minutes or so and, when this is chewed thoroughly, deposit it onto a green leaf. Local etiquette demands that men chew one another's kava, particularly in the case of honored guests. When sufficient kava is ready, a virgin boy places several mouthfuls of the chewed pulp (three is an average) onto the burlap-like stipule sheath of a coconut frond that he and a partner hold taut. Someone pours water slowly onto the masticated kava that the boy squeezes and mixes as the drink strains into a half coconut shell cup placed below the strainer. This first straining is "the body" of the kava. Drinkers, later in the evening, may also restrain used kava pulp, this second drink called the "spirit" or "shadow" of the kava. In Bislama, used kava pulp is called *makas*, a word that derives from "bagasse," the remnant sugarcane fiber produced in sugar refining. Tannese occasionally mix kava in oblong bowls named "canoes"; this method of preparation is reflective of Polynesian practice. These bowls were in more common use before the twentieth century.

In northern parts of Vanuatu (e.g., Ambae, Pentecost, Maewo, the Banks and Torres Islands), men grate and grind kava on cylindrical coral abrading stones. Holding the coral abrader in one hand, they grate kava root against it with the other, allowing root particles to drop down onto a wooden dish. Men next infuse this ground root in water, holding a strainer several feet in the air above a half coconut shell cup. Kava, cascading down into the cup below, thus acquires a head of froth. In some communities, drinkers occasionally do not infuse grated kava in water. Instead, they drink undiluted juices that they manage to wring from the ground root.

In the Admiralty Islands of Papua New Guinea and on Pohnpei (and formerly on neighboring Kosrae) men prepare kava by placing roots on large, flat basaltic anvils, and pounding them with water-worn hammer stones. On Pohnpei, three or four men rhythmically pound kava making the anvil stone ring with bell-like tones. Heard widely, these ringing stones let people know that kava soon will be ready. Different families and villages own rights to particular kava-pounding rhythms. Kava makers infuse pounded kava in wooden bowls (*tanoa*) or, nowadays, plastic buckets. Finally, they strain kava infusions through the green and slimy inner-bark of *H. tiliaceus*. This bark gives Pohnpei kava, distinctive within the Pacific, a notably viscous character. Use of green bark to strain kava, rather than dried as is the case elsewhere, may be a modern innovation dating to around 1915 (Riesenberg, 1968).

Kava preparation today in bars on Pohnpei, and also in Port Vila's *nakamals* – which feature green kava – relies on various sorts of mechanical grinders, some hand-cranked

and some motorized, to process the rootstock. Bartenders infuse ground kava in recep-
tacles such as plastic buckets and bowls or enamel basins, and they strain the drink
through whatever material is at hand including women's nylon hose. Bars serve the
drink in glasses, bowls, enamel cups, or traditional coconut half shells, typically sold as
"large" or "small."

In contemporary Fiji, Samoa, and Tonga, producers process dried kava by pounding
this in makeshift mortars (hollow tree stumps or metal pipes) using a variety of wooden
or metal pestles. Instead of filtering kava grounds from the bowl after infusion – the
traditional technique – kava makers today may first wrap powdered kava in scraps of
cloth and then squeeze this bundle in water to leach out kavalactones without getting
grounds into the drink.

Human and plant physiology inform kava consumption practice. People, for
example, typically drink kava on an empty stomach – often at dusk – presumably so
kavalactone molecules will more easily pass through stomach membranes. Almost
everywhere, people down cups of kava all at once. Kava rarely is sipped and savored,
perhaps because of its typically bitter or earthy flavor, and also because of longstanding
tradition. Immediately after drinking, a person may eat a small meal. As kava continues
to be absorbed into the body, it dulls appetite. Depending on drunken comportment
etiquette, and also on the concentration of the drink, imbibers in some societies will
continue to joke and talk while they eat and drink additional rounds. In Fiji, Samoa,
Tonga, and northern Vanuatu, kava consumers engage in lively conversation, sometimes joking and singing, and may prepare several bowls of kava to share during an
evening. In other places, all conversation and noise cease as drinkers concentrate on the
drug's effects. In southern Vanuatu and in Pohnpei, for example, people believe that
noise and bright light prevent or spoil their intoxication. Everyone falls silent in order
to "listen" to the kava.

Preparation and consumption, particularly in Polynesian societies as well as Fiji, is
intricately choreographed by a complicated etiquette (Churchill, 1916; Mead, 1930;
Lester, 1941). Participants sit in a circle around often beautifully carved kava bowls,
their position within this circle dictated by their relative social and political status.
Servers, who carry coconut shell cups from kava bowl to drinker, walk and present the
cup in a ritually stylized fashion. In Fiji, participants in kava circles clap three times
after each man drinks. Typically, drinking order serves as a model of chiefly hierarchy
within the region, with men who hold higher status titles drinking both first and last.
In Samoa, for example, the highest ranking chief (*matai*) drinks first, followed by the
highest-ranking orator (or "talking chief," *tulafale*), and so on down the ranks to untitled
younger men, with one higher ranking chief bringing up the rear. Elsewhere, kava
preparation is less formalized. Men gather at the end of the day and chat and gossip as
they prepare kava in bowls or plastic buckets that they will drink together with no
particular regard for etiquette or order of service.

Patterns of kava consumption correlate with age, gender, and status differences. As
noted above, women in many societies had fewer rights and opportunities to consume
kava than did men. Such taboos recently have decayed somewhat, particularly in urban
centers. For a man, changing access to kava reflects his passage through life. On Tanna,
for example, where men and boys gather to prepare and drink kava daily on circular
forest clearings just out of sight from hamlets and villages, young boys, still uncircumcised,
follow along and participate as observers only. After boys are circumcised (between ages
six and twelve or so), they begin chewing kava root to prepare this for their elders

to drink. Boys also have the duty of mixing and squeezing the pulp in their hands, infusing it in cold water so long as they remain virgins. Sexually active youths continue to chew kava for their elders, but may no longer touch chewed root. Older men who have sons to prepare their kava sit about gossiping and politicking until their kava is ready. Local leaders generally are the first to drink while less important and younger men follow behind.

Tannese patterns of kava preparation and consumption thus track important gender, age, and political differences on the island. The plant and the drink command similar symbolic importance wherever kava is known and used. Kava continues to be a key part of Pacific Island society – in subsistence and commercial economies, in political arenas, in religious ritual, old and new, in folk pharmacy, and in smoothing the course of everyday life.

References

Aloha Seed & Herb (n.d.) *Kava-for-Health.com* (website).

Arno, A. (1992) *The World is Talk: Conflict and Communication on a Fijian Island*, Albex, Norwood, NJ.

Baal, J.V. (1966) *Dema*, Martinus Nijhoff, Leiden.

Beaglehole, E. and Beaglehole, P. (1941) *Pangai Village in Tonga*, Memoirs of the Polynesian Society, No. 18, The Polynesian Society, Wellington, NZ.

Brunton, R. (1989) *The Abandoned Narcotic: Kava and Cultural Instability in Melanesia*, Cambridge University Press, Cambridge.

Burrows, E.G. (1936) *Ethnology of Futuna*, Bulletin No. 138, Bernice P. Bishop Museum Press, Honolulu.

Capell, A. (1960) *Anthropology and Linguistics of Futuna-Aniwa*, Oceania Linguistic Monograph No. 5, University of Sydney, Sydney.

Churchill, W. (1916) *Samoan Kava Custom*, Holmes Anniversary, Washington DC.

Clunie, F. (1986) *Yalo i Viti*, Fiji Museum, Suva.

Cowling, W. (1988) Kava and tradition in Tonga. In J. Prescott and G. McCall (eds), *Kava Use and Abuse in Australia and the South Pacific*, Monograph No. 5, National Drug and Alcohol Research Centre, University of New South Wales, Sydney.

Firth, R. (1970) *Rank and Religion in Tikopia*, George Allen and Unwin, London, pp. 199–232.

Furst, P.T. (1972) *Flesh of the Gods: The Ritual Use of Hallucinogens*, Praeger, New York.

Gaillot, M. (1962) Le rite du kava Futunien. *Études Mélanésiennes* (4th ser.), 14–17, 95–105.

Gifford, E.W. (1929) *Tongan Society*, Bulletin No. 61, Bernice P. Bishop Museum Press, Honolulu.

Haddon, A.C. (1916) Kava drinking in New Guinea. *Man*, 16, 145–152.

Hammer Corporation (n.d.) *Black Fire*, Hammer Corp., Atlanta.

Hocart, A.M. (1929) *Lau Islands, Fiji*, Bulletin No. 62, Bernice P. Bishop Museum, Honolulu.

Holmes, L.D. (1961) The Samoan kava ceremony: its forms and functions. *Science of Man*, 1, 46–51.

Kilham, C. (1996) *Kava: Medicine Hunting in Paradise*, Park Street Press, Rochester, VT.

Knauft, B. (1987) Managing sex and anger: tobacco and kava use among the Gebusi of Papua New Guinea. In L. Lindstrom (ed.), *Drugs in Western Pacific Societies: Relations of Substance*, University Press of America, Lanham, MD, pp. 73–98.

Lamboll, R. (1989) *Kava in Vanuatu: The Advent of a Cash Crop*, Internal Report, Vanuatu Government Department of Agriculture, Port Vila.

Landtman, G. (1927) *The Kiwai Papuans of British New Guinea*, Macmillan, London.

Layard, J. (1942) *Stone Men of Malakula*, Chatto and Windus, London.

Lebot, V. (1989) L'histoire du kava commence par sa découverte. *Journal de la Société des Océanistes*, **88/89**, 89–114.

Lebot, V. and Lévesque (1989) The origin and distribution of kava (*Piper methysticum* Forst. f. and *Piper wichmannii* C. DC., Piperaceae): A phytochemical approach. *Allertonia*, 5, 223–280.

Lebot, V., Merlin, M. and Lindstrom, L. (1992) *Kava: The Pacific Drug*, Yale University Press, New Haven CT.

Lester, R.H. (1941) Kava drinking in Viti Levu, Fiji. *Oceania*, 12, 97–124.

Linden, L. (2000) Second kava DUI case dismissed. *Oakland Tribune*, 26 December.

Lindstrom, L. (1980) Spitting on Tanna. *Oceania*, 50, 228–234.

Lindstrom, L. (1987) Drunkenness and gender on Tanna, Vanuatu. In L. Lindstrom (ed.), *Drugs in Western Pacific Societies: Relations of Substance*, University Press of America, Lanham, MD, pp. 99–118.

McGrath, T.B. (1973) *Sakau* in towm, *Sarawi* in towm. *Oceania*, 44, 64–67.

Mead, M. (1930) *Social Organization of Manu'a*, Bulletin No. 76, Bernice P. Bishop Museum Press, Honolulu.

Newell, W.H. (1947) Kava ceremony in Tonga. *Journal of the Polynesian Society*, 56, 364–417.

Oliver, D.L. (1974) *Ancient Tahitian Society*, Australian National University Press, Canberra.

Reichel-Dolmatoff, G. (1972) The cultural context of an Aboriginal hallucinogen: *Banisteriopsis caapi*. In P.T. Furst (ed.), *Flesh of the Gods: The Ritual Use of Hallucinogens*, Praeger, New York, pp. 84–113.

Riesenberg, S.H. (1968) *The Native Polity of Ponape*, Smithsonian Institution Press, Washington, DC.

Rivers, W.H.R. (1914) *The History of the Melanesian Society*, Cambridge University Press, Cambridge.

Roth, G.K. (1953) *Fijian Way of Life*, Oxford University Press, Melbourne.

Schübel, K. (1924) Chemistry and pharmacology of kawa-kawa (*Piper methysticum*). *Journal of the Society of Chemical Industry*, 43, 766B.

Schultes, R.E. and Hofmann, A. (1979) *Plants of the Gods*, MacGraw-Hill, New York.

Siméoni, P. (2002) D'oùvient le nikawa? *Journal de la Société des Océanistes*, 14/15, 209–222.

Singh, Y.N. (1992) Kava: an overview. *Journal of Ethnopharmacology*, 37, 13–45.

Singh, Y.N. and Blumenthal, M.A. (1997) Kava: an overview. Distribution, mythology, botany, culture, chemistry, and pharmacology of the South Pacific's most revered herb. *HerbalGram*, 39, 33–45.

Steinmetz, E.F. (1960) *Kava Kava* (Piper methysticum*): Famous Drug Plant of the South Sea Islands*, Level Press, San Francisco.

Thompson, L.M. (1940) *Southern Lau, Fiji: An Ethnography*, Bulletin No. 162, Bernice P. Bishop Museum Press, Honolulu.

Titcomb, M. (1948) Kava in Hawaii. *Journal of the Polynesian Society*, 57, 105–171.

Toren, C. (1999) *Mind, Materiality, and History: Explorations in Fijian Ethnography*, Routledge, London.

Turner, J.W. (1986) The water of life: kava ritual and the logic of sacrifice. *Ethnology*, 25, 203–214.

Wasson, R.G. (1980) *The Wondrous Mushroom: Mycolatry in Mesoamerica*, McGraw-Hill, NewYork.

Williamson, R.W. (1939) *Essays in Polynesian Ethnology*, Cambridge University Press, Cambridge.

3 Kava: Production, Marketing and Quality Assurance

Yadhu N. Singh

Introduction

As a crop, kava is well suited to the farming methods that have been developed by the Pacific Islanders. Its flexible cultivation requirements and its ability to thrive in the shade and in traditional multicrop gardens make it a preferred crop for the subsistence way of life prevalent in that part of the world. Like most other important Pacific crops, it is asexually propagated. Cloning of a single cultivar by using stem cuttings results in a population of genetically identical progeny. Thus, by choosing healthy and robust planting material and using good farming practices, high yields of a superior crop can usually be assured. This chapter discusses: methods of cultivation and harvesting; measures that ensure high quality products; and, the marketing and economics of this important Oceanic crop.

Production

Since its domestication about 3000 years ago, kava has continuously been cultivated in the Pacific Islands for its cultural, social, medical, and magico-religious use. Thus a large body of traditional knowledge concerning its production has accumulated. However, with the recent growth of the commercial market, both in the Pacific and around the world, more efficient and large-scale cultivation and planting techniques are being developed.

Cultivation

Site selection

The choice of a suitable site is of paramount importance to the success of the crop. For the young plant to develop properly, it should be sheltered from the sun and the wind. Thus kava grows well in traditional multicrop gardens where it is partly shaded by taller crops such as bananas, papayas, and tapioca (manioc). Exposure to the sun speeds up moisture loss and makes the plant prone to wilting. Prevailing southeasterly tradewinds may bend stems and branches and damage rootstock, causing them to crack or break, and thus encourage disease in the plant. The plant also requires high average temperatures (20–35 °C), high humidity (about 70% or higher), and average annual precipitation of over 200 cm.

Kava grows best in fertile, well-drained, loose soil which should not be allowed to dry out. Soils prone to water-logging should be avoided as this can inhibit growth and lead to root rot. Best yields are obtained in silica-clay soils with a pH of 5.5–6.5, high humus content, and a physical structure conducive to the free circulation of air and moisture. For this reason, kava is often planted on gently sloping land because drainage is better than in valley floors, which run the risk of water-logging. However, mounding up of soil into ridges can be employed on flat land gardens.

Planting material

As discussed in Chapter 4, there is a substantial diversity in the kava cultivars in the Pacific. According to Lebot *et al.* (1997), the number of different cultivars identified in the various island groups varies, with over 80 in Vanuatu, about 14 in Hawaii, 12 in Fiji, 8 in Tonga, 5 in Samoa, 4 in Papua New Guinea, 3 in Wallis and Futuna and also in French Polynesia, and 2 in Pohnpei. As kava does not produce viable seeds, there is no possibility of cross pollination to create new cultivars. However, a process of selection by farmers over many generations for kava plants with the most desirable characteristics for personal and ceremonial use has resulted in a diversity of cultivars.

Experienced growers know that one of the most important decisions in producing quality kava is the selection of the planting material. The cutting should come from a vigorous and healthy plant of a desirable cultivar, that is, one with good drinking characteristics. The cutting should be carefully inspected to ensure it is free from disease and infestation. It should be from the more rot-resistant woody mid to lower portions of the stem, rather than from the soft upper stem which is prone to rot and does not develop vigorous roots and shoots. Also lateral branches should not be used as they will produce plants with horizontal stems.

The normal method of propagation is to use cuttings of one to four nodes in length, although the process may vary. Either shoots or stem cuttings can be used, and cuttings are either planted first in a nursery or directly planted in the gardens.

In vivo *propagation*

Tissue culture techniques are being investigated for kava to assist in clonal propagation, germplasm conservation, and plant improvement. Experience with a number of *Piper* species has shown that tissue culture initiation is severely hampered by a high incidence of bacterial and fungal infection (Fitchet, 1990). Bhat *et al.* (1995) have reported that after decontamination, micropropagation of *P. betle*, *P. nigrum*, and *P. longum* was successfully carried out. However, decontamination of kava, which appears to have a high innoculum of bacteria and fungi, was not achieved, and when it was effective, only fungal contaminants were eliminated in the majority of cases.

These problems with decontamination of explants has greatly inhibited the development of a kava micropropagation system (Taylor and Taufa, 1998). Once the decontamination procedures have been resolved, there are several other aspects that need to be evaluated before a kava micropropagation system becomes feasible. The shoot multiplication stage needs to be developed to make the system commercially viable and the rooting of the generated shoots must not be a problem. Tissue culture plantlets should transfer to the soil without significant delay in growth or losses in plants. Finally and significantly, analysis of the established plants must be carried out to ensure that the tissue culture process has not adversely affected the kavalactone composition and content.

False kava

A possible threat to the quality and reputation of kava is the recent inadvertent introduction of so-called "false kava" into all major kava growing regions of the Pacific. The plants resemble the genuine kava but lack the kavalactones and the distinct kava odor. The main false kava species are *P. auritum* and *P. aduncum*. A fuller discussion on this topic can be found in Chapter 4.

Since the false kava species closely resemble the genuine variety, care must be taken to exclude them during the selection of the planting material, although this is not a problem with experienced kava planters in the Pacific.

Direct planting

Traditionally, kava stem cuttings are planted directly in the field. A handful of one- and two-node cuttings can be planted together in an approximately 30 cm diameter circle. Alternatively, four- to six-node cuttings are planted vertically or semi-vertically with several nodes buried in the soil. Sometimes cuttings are rooted in loose soil before planting. Often the cuttings are planted and covered with a layer of mulch to retain moisture since adequate moisture is critical for the shoot and root development.

Kava should be planted out in the field as early in the rainy season as possible. In intercropping situations, where intercropping is used to provide shade and wind shelter to the young kava plants, some delay is advisable to permit the intercrop to become established before the kava is planted. A lead time of about two to three months is usually required. However, delaying the kava planting for too long may result in the dry season setting in while the kava is still in its delicate growing stages.

With the increased demand for kava both in the Pacific and abroad, the direct planting method is proving to be less efficient for the following reasons. Moist conditions and shade are essential for developing shoots and roots and young plants. However, extensive watering required for the direct planting method can be more costly and labor intensive and providing shade against the tropical sun is more difficult in the fields than in the nursery. The desired spacing is difficult to achieve with direct planting because not all cuttings or nodes may germinate and produce plants. Furthermore, weed competition with young kava seedlings is a problem that requires considerable labor input and can slow down the growth of the young kava plant.

Nurseries and transplanting

The shortage of planting material caused by the expansion in production during the late 1990s stimulated interest in kava nurseries in many countries, because of the better germination of cuttings and higher survival rate of plants when transplanted to the field.

The nursery should be located on well-drained land to avoid being waterlogged or flooded during heavy rains, but with easy access to water for irrigation during dry periods. The soil for the nursery can be derived from rich topsoil, sand and compost, and other media such as potting soil. Heavy clay should be avoided as it can become too wet and this encourages the development of fungus in the plants.

Kava requires a high level of nutrient supply for good performance, although many kava growers may not make a deliberate effort to boost the native fertility of the soil. Inorganic fertilizer use can be of substantial benefit to the kava crop. At the time of direct planting or on transplanting, complete NPK (sodium, phosphorus, potassium) fertilizer (typically 12:12:20) is mixed at the bottom of each hole or planting site. At four months after planting, urea (with 45% nitrogen) is applied. Subsequent fertilizer may be applied every six months, depending on observed nutrient deficiencies. However, kava is sensitive to contact with inorganic fertilizers; thus direct contact with the roots should be avoided. The roots are most likely to be damaged if band or spot application of fertilizer is employed. Instead, it should be evenly spread a little distance away from the roots.

Cuttings with one or two nodes from woody mature stems, two to three years old, are laid lengthwise in rows with the bud scars facing up, and spaced about 10 cm apart to make it easier for digging up and transplanting. A layer of soil about 3 cm deep is gently laid over the cuttings before thoroughly watering the rows. A more labor-saving method involves using a whole lower kava stem with many nodes and bud scars. However, the roots from adjoining nodes may become tangled and are likely to be damaged when being dug up and transplanted in the fields.

Alternatively, seedlings may be grown in "polypots" or "polybags," which are strong black plastic nursery bags, and are available in a variety of sizes. Polypots are commonly used in commercial nurseries, and measure about 7.5 cm in diameter and 30 cm high. The cuttings, usually with one or two bud scars, are planted horizontally in the bag. Polypots are popular because they keep the roots from growing together and reduce the risk of root damage during transplantation.

Transplanting is normally done when the seedlings are about 30 cm tall; they can avoid competition from weeds, the moisture conditions in the fields are favorable, and the land has been properly prepared. The plants are gradually acclimatized to direct sunlight before they are removed from the nursery. After transplanting, sufficient shade and water are provided for the plants to become established and to grow well in the fields.

Cropping

The natural habitat for kava is dense rainforest under the shade of large trees and shrubs, and it is still grown in association with other crops. Experience and research have shown that intercropping has major advantages. Above all, it can reduce or inhibit the spread of disease among kava plants whereas monocropping can encourage it.

In intercropping the crops are changed over the growth cycle of the kava. When the kava plants are small, intercrops which provide shade, such as taro and pigeon peas, are helpful. Later, when the kava needs more sunlight, intercrops like sweet potatoes and peanuts which provide good ground cover and thus reduce weed growth and retain soil moisture are useful. Sometimes, kava is grown with a variety of vegetables such as tomatoes, Chinese cabbage (a variety of bok choy), cabbage, capsicum, and eggplant. However, kava is vulnerable to many diseases and insects associated with these vegetables, and thus intercropping with them should be avoided. Planting kava with ginger is also inadvisable as the same kinds of nematodes which attack ginger can also attack kava. Intercropping kava with coconut trees is common and a natural association in the Pacific. The coconut trees provide excellent and extensive shade. However, they have shallow, fibrous roots that extend well beyond the canopy of the fronds. These roots compete with kava for water and nutrients making its harvesting difficult. Sufficient spacing between rows of coconut trees and kava plants, about 4–5 m, usually avoids root competition.

Crop care

Weed competition is a major problem in kava production and traditionally hoeing and manual removal have been the major methods of weeding. However, weeding hoes should not be used too close to the plants as serious damage can be caused to the surface roots, to the adventitious roots from the stem and to the young shoots. Recently, herbicides have been used for weed control; however, there are important reasons why they should be avoided, at least at this point in time. Not enough research has been done on the appropriate types and amount of herbicides for kava production. It is also known that the kava plant is very sensitive to some herbicides, resulting in wilting even when used some distance from the plant.

Although kava cultivation is recommended only in high rainfall areas, it does not preclude use of locations with a marked dry season, provided that the drought does not last too long, or irrigation is readily available. The plants are especially sensitive to drought stress and water logging during the first six months. Shading the plants and using windbreaks in windy areas throughout the life of the plants will reduce moisture loss.

Each node of the lateral branches could sprout roots when they come in contact with the soil. This is allowed to occur without interference for the first 10–11 months of growth. At about one year the lateral branches are trimmed just beyond the root growth from the last node and at the point where a new shoot has sprouted. The trimming of lateral roots encourages the development of the root system rather than the shoots which is preferable since the roots are the more valuable harvested plant part.

Diseases and pests

The major constraints to kava production in the South Pacific are due to various diseases and pests. Of these, a dieback disease is the most serious (Davis *et al.*, 1996). Other diseases appear to have a lesser impact on plant productivity. Some insects and other pests have been shown to attack, though the kava weevil borer is the only insect recorded as causing serious damage.

Dieback disease

The first report of this disease was made in Fiji by Parham (1935) who described a wilt disease that in some instances caused major sections of the crop to be abandoned or destroyed. Later, it was found to occur in other kava-growing countries of Samoa, Tonga, and Vanuatu. Plant pathologists in Fiji have estimated that dieback disease causes annual crop losses of up to 60% (Brown, 1989; MAFF, 2001).

The dieback disease is characterized by a black rotting of stems, which may eventually disintegrate (Figure 3.1). New shoots often arise from the base of affected plants, and the cycles of dieback and regrowth are repeated until the whole plant eventually dies. If left unchecked, entire plantations may be destroyed by the disease. The infected plant will first show symptoms of the disease on its leaves. They begin by developing yellow veins and yellow and green patterns, gradually causing the leaves to become crinkled and puckered. The stems below the infected leaves show brown streaks and/or patches

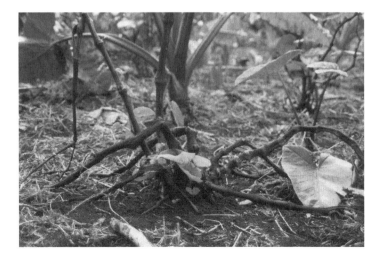

Figure 3.1 Symptoms of kava dieback disease caused by cucumber mosaic cucumovirus (CMV). Severe dieback of stems and an attempt at regrowth. Note the multicropping of kava with *Colocasia* sp. Photo provided by Dr Richard Davis.

of rot in the vascular and surrounding tissues. Sometimes, internal discolored areas also occur in stems at soil level and in the roots. After three to four weeks the symptoms are noticeable externally.

Pares and co-workers (1992) showed that the cucumber mosaic virus (CMV) was present in leaves showing mosaic, mottled, and chlorotic symptoms. Subsequently, Davis and colleagues (1996) found that CMV was widely distributed in kava plants in all major kava-producing countries. They also showed that the symptoms of the dieback disease developed on plants inoculated with CMV, usually within three to four weeks after leaf symptoms first became visible. It is now accepted that the CMV is the main causative agent for the kava dieback disease. The disease is also aggravated by plant-sucking pests such as the leaf miner and aphids which create entry in the cells for the CMV, and by infections from soil borne nematodes, fungi, and bacteria.

No adequate control measures have been developed against the dieback disease. The most effective precautions appear to be adequate spacing between plants and intercropping. Adequate field sanitation, use of virus free planting material, and pruning out of diseased plants are used effectively in many countries.

Nematodes

The most current information on nematodes in kava was obtained by Orton Williams (1980) who conducted extensive surveys throughout the South Pacific. He identified the following parasitic plant nematodes on kava.

Spiral nematodes (*Helicotylenchus rotundicauda* Sher, *H. dihystera* (Cobb) Sher, *H. multicinctus* (Cobb) Golden, and *H. mucronatus* Siddiqi). This genus is the most commonly encountered nematode on kava in the South Pacific. Almost all plantings were infested by at least one of the species.

Reniform nematode (*Rotylenchulus reniformis* Linford and Oliveira) was present in 50–70% of the kava plantings in Fiji, Tonga, and Samoa.

Root-knot nematodes (*Meloidogyne javanica* (Treub.) Chitwood, *M. incognita* (Kofoid and White) Chitwood, and *M. arenaria* (Neal) (Chitwood)) are widespread throughout the region, and roots affected by these nematodes were often encountered.

G.R. Stirling, who conducted a survey of nematodes associated with kava on the island of Tongatapu in Tonga (Davis and Brown, 1999), concluded that there is every likelihood that plant parasitic nematodes, particularly *Meloidogyne* spp., *R. reniformis* and *R. similis*, cause economic damage to kava crops. These nematodes are all serious pathogens of other Pacific crops, and specific symptoms of *Meloidogyne* spp. and *R. similis* were observed on kava roots.

In pathogenicity tests conducted by Davis and Brown (1999) with *M. javanica*, where kava and tomato plants were inoculated under identical conditions, the innoculum levels used (10^5 eggs per plant) were sufficient to kill the tomato plants. The extent of root gall or lump development in kava plants was minor and would not have been expected to significantly reduce plant growth.

Fungal diseases

Almost 20 fungi have been found to be associated with disease symptoms in kava, although in many instances pathogenicity tests to prove a causal relationship between the presence of the fungus and the disease symptoms have not been undertaken.

Anthracnose: Symptoms associated with the presence of one or more species of *Colletotrium*, particularly *C. gloeosporioides* (Penz.) Sacc., are common throughout the main kava-producing countries (Kumar *et al.*, 1985; Brown and Minchinton, 1989). The pathogens cause small (3 cm^2 in area or less) irregularly shaped dark lesions on the stems. The disease appears to have little effect on productivity. The disease is effectively controlled by the use of dithiocarbamate fungicidal sprays. Wider spacing between plants and intercropping has also lowered incidence of the disease.

Sphaerulina leaf spots: These usually are less than 1 cm in diameter and initially black in color with their centers turning white enclosed by dark margin in mature lesions. The disease is thought to be caused by the Ascomycete *Sphaerulina* spp. (Gerlach, 1988). The disease is most prevalent in a warm, moist environment such as that of Samoa and is less common in the cooler and drier climate of Tonga.

Sclerotium rolfsii: This often forms a white mycelium and pale yellow-brown spherical sclerotia on the external surface of kava roots and stem base. Some authors (e.g., Singh and Nambiar, 1988) consider the fungus to be pathogenic on kava. However, in pathogenicity tests, where 300 sclerotia were placed adjacent to roots of potted kava plants, the fungus killed only those plants whose roots had been severely injured prior to inoculation (Davis and Brown, 1999). Thus, *S. rolfsii* may play a role as a secondary pathogen of kava roots.

Bacteria

Soft-rotting bacteria of the genus *Erwinia* are commonly found in kava but *Erwinia* spp. were pathogenic only to uninjured kava (Butler, 1973, 1974). However, Heinlein and co-workers (1984) were unable to demonstrate that *E. carotovora* (Jones) Bergy was pathogenic on kava. Pathogenicity tests by Davis and Brown (1999) showed that

E. carotovora pv. *carotovora* (Jones) Dye 1923 produced a black soft rot when inoculated onto injured (but not uninjured) kava stems. The symptoms were similar to those of the black soft rot characteristic of kava dieback disease. Thus, the bacterium was capable of killing kava plants which were already damaged, suggesting that this species may act as a secondary parasite under certain circumstances.

Insects and other pests

A few attempts have been made to quantify the damage caused on kava by insects and other pests but surveys on the effects by individual pests are severely lacking.

Kava weevil borer (*Elytroteinous subtruncatus* Fairm.) is the only insect reported as causing serious damage to kava plants. Surveys in Tonga in the late 1970s estimated that the weevil borer caused 28% damage to kava crops (Fakalata, 1981; Fakalata and Langi, 1983). The female weevils bore into the stems of kava and lay eggs. The larvae hatch and tunnel inside the stems causing them to become weakened and prone to infection by secondary soft-rotting fungi and bacteria. The weevil is best controlled by use of insecticides. It is recommended to paint the weevil hole with Sevin, or to spray the infected plants with Diazinon, Furadan, or similar insecticide. Careful selection of planting material is also important in weevil control.

Aphids are plant fluid feeding pests of kava. *Aphis gossypii* is the most common found on kava in Tonga. Extremely large colonies can become established, especially during dry weather. However, the most damaging aspect of aphid infestation is their role as a vector of CMV, the cause of kava dieback.

Mites are small plant fluid sucking pests. The two major species which have been identified are the two-spotted mite (*Tetranychus urticae* Koch.) and the bulb mite (*Rhizoglyphus echinopus* Fumouze and Robin). In dry conditions, large mite colonies can build up on kava plants, causing significant damage in nurseries and in the field. Severely affected leaves become chlorotic, curled, and necrotic on the margins.

Mealy bugs (*Planococcus* spp.) are also plant fluid sucking insects which sometimes attack kava aerial parts and roots. Severe infestation can lead to defoliation, and in the case of root infestation, to a general unsightly plant appearance.

Army worms (*Spodoptera* spp.) can cause damage in kava nurseries and sometimes in the fields where they feed directly on the foliage. The pest can cause complete plant defoliation.

Giant African land snail (*Achatina fulica* Bowditch) can damage kava crops if it transfers from its normal diet of detritus to the kava plant. The snail has so far been detected in Fiji, Samoa, and Vanuatu, but not in Tonga.

Harvesting and Processing

Harvesting and yields

Harvesting and post-harvest handling account for about half of the labor involved in kava production. Particular attention needs to be given to harvesting, handling, drying, and storage since these operations have a major impact on the quality of kava and its price.

Kava is normally ready for harvest after three to four years of growth, but the harvest may be delayed sometimes to allow for the plant, especially the rootstock, to become larger and to acquire a higher kavalactone content. In general, kavalactone content increases with the age of the plant. However, some research indicates that kavalactone content depends more on the type of soil, the availability of water and nutrients for plant growth, and the particular kava cultivar than on the age of the plant (Lebot *et al.*, 1997).

Harvesting is done manually with hand tools as mechanical harvesting is non-existent. The process begins with the removal of the stems about 30–60 cm from the ground level. Then a hole is dug around the base of the plant to free the crown and the proximal portions of the root. The depth and extent of digging depends on how large and submerged the crown is, which itself may depend on the extent of mounding or earthing-up that was done while the crop was growing. If the digging is insufficiently thorough, some of the valuable roots may be left behind in the soil when the crop is pulled out. As a result of these requirements, harvesting kava can be a slow, tedious, and laborious operation. An average worker normally harvests only about three to four plants per hour.

The marketable yield of kava consists of the crown and the larger roots attached to it. The typical yield from a three- to four-year-old plant would be about 10–11 kg fresh weight. About 80% of this would be comprised of the crown proper with the rest being made up of attached roots. Under very favorable cultivation conditions, yields of up to 50 kg plants are possible and in rare instances, fresh harvests of 100 kg or more from a single plant have been reported (Lebot *et al.*, 1997).

Processing

After harvesting, the stages in processing of the material are: washing, cutting and sorting, chipping or peeling, drying, storage, powdering, sieving, and packing.

Washing

The yield is carefully and thoroughly washed in water to remove the soil particles and attached debris. Thus easy access to sufficient water is imperative as moving the bulky, freshly harvested material to a water source can pose a problem and may also cause damage to the kava. If the washing is done in a tank, a small amount of soap may be used, but care should be taken to remove all of it by the end of the washing process.

Cutting, peeling, and sorting

The kava is now ready, with some exceptions, to be cut up, peeled if desired, and sorted according to the plant parts before drying. The valuable thin long roots are not cut up before drying (Figure 3.2). The basal stems (the first 20–30 cm of the stems) are removed, peeled, and cut into pieces. The roots are removed from the rootstock, peeled, then cut into small pieces. Each part of the harvested kava is kept separate as the kava-lactones content and hence the market value for each plant part is different. For this reason, kava buyers both for the local drinking market and for export require that the product be separated into peels from the roots and crown, chips from the root, chips from the crown, and chips from the base stem, representing the decreasing order of kavalactone content.

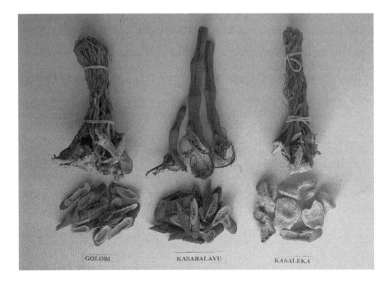

Figure 3.2 Rootlets, roots, and chips from two white varieties (*golobi* and *kasaleka*) and a black variety (*kasabalavu*) of kava from Fiji. Photo by Yatesh Singh.

Drying

After the kava has been cut, peeled, and sorted, it is subjected to drying. The drying process should always be done on raised platforms, never on the ground, to avoid mixing with soil and dirt, insects, grass, and other foreign matter. For a long time, sun drying has been done by spreading out the kava on corrugated iron sheets which reflect additional heat. Sometimes, kava may be seen spread on the metal roofs of houses, if no rain is expected, as with rain water the kava will get wet and become discolored or rot. Black plastic is also used and drying racks made from fine mesh chicken wire are becoming popular. The rate of drying depends on the water content of the kava, the relative humidity of the air, and wind currents blowing over the kava. As the weather is very variable in the tropics, and where large amounts of kava are being processed for commercial markets, newer drying technologies are being developed. For instance, drying racks may be placed inside makeshift structures which are covered on all sides by plastic sheets designed to keep out the rain and also to trap the solar heat. More permanent kava drying sheds with clear plastic roofs and vented walls made of wood are becoming more common.

The initial water content of the fresh material is about 80%, and this needs to be reduced to about 12% or less to minimize deterioration due to rotting and fungal attack during handling and storage. The dried material is checked for moisture content by bending a root – if it is sufficiently dry, it will break, but will be flexible and merely bend if it needs further drying.

Storage

After drying, the chips, peels, roots, etc., are packaged separately, usually in 25 kg woven polypropylene sacks (similar to gunny sacks) which allow some degree of aeration.

Kava, like other dry agricultural products, is hygroscopic. In the high humidity of the tropics, this can lead to rapid deterioration of the material and development of fungus and a mouldy smell, resulting in loss of quality and value of the product. Hence, the moisture level in dried kava needs to be continuously monitored and, if necessary, redried, although multiple drying can also cause deterioration in quality. Thus, it is advisable that for best results the storage period be kept as short as possible and the kava used soon after it is processed.

Powdering

Kava destined for the pharmaceutical industry abroad and some for recreational use both locally and abroad is usually not processed further in the producing countries, but exported as chips, peels, roots, etc. It is stored temporarily in a dry location until it is shipped out. Traditionally, kava was pounded or chewed before the beverage was prepared. While chewing has virtually disappeared except in Vanuatu (and Wallis and Futuna), mechanical pounding is still widely practiced as many of the drinkers in the South Pacific contend that kava powder produced by mechanical grinding is usually discolored and of inferior quality. There is, however, no scientific evidence for this claim.

Mechanical pounding or grinding is a protracted process. After a batch has been pounded or ground, a high proportion of the batch remains coarse, so that after sieving out of the fine particles the residue is returned for further pounding or grinding. The powdered kava that results is packed into plastic containers or bags, sealed, and sent out for domestic use or to the export market.

In Vanuatu, where kava beverage for consumption is prepared immediately after harvesting, meat grinders are often used to pulverize the fresh roots. The pulp is then suspended in water, sieved, and drunk right away. In some locations, chewing or pieces of rock and coral may be used for grating the kava, common methods before the advent of mechanical devices (see Chapter 2).

Industrial processing

Unpowdered rootstock and dry stumps are now exported in large quantities for use by laboratories overseas. The product is, especially in the United States, then processed into hydro-alcoholic extracts that are partially soluble in water and alcohol. Alternatively, extraction is done using other organic solvents, such as acetone and chloroform. With the expanding kava demand for pharmaceutical preparations (before the liver toxicity controversy), more refined extraction processes were being developed. These processes can produce a wide range of industrial products, including freeze-dried extracts from a filtered macerate, an essential oil by distilling leaves with water, an extract of active kavalactones isolated using volatile solvents, and spray-drying of enriched fresh juices. Spray-dried hydrosoluble powder is a promising product that could be locally produced in the islands and then exported.

The American Herbal Products Association (AHPA), which was founded in 1983 to promote the responsible commerce of products that contain herbs, is now in the United States the national trade association and voice of the herbal products industry. It is comprised of companies doing business as growers, manufacturers, and marketers of herbs and herbal products. AHPA has been active in creating standards for herbal products, and has done so by drawing on the expertise of its members and their extensive experience.

In the past few years (1999–2001), AHPA's Botanical Extracts Committee has developed three documents intended to provide guidelines for various issues encountered in the manufacture, labeling, and sale of herbal extracts, including kava. The first, *Guidance for the Manufacture and Sale of Bulk Botanical Extracts*, contains definitions of extract terminology as well as descriptions of the most common extract manufacturing processes, and also discusses quality control issues and offers guidance for bulk product labeling. The stated goal of this document is to reduce the confusion that exists in the marketplace about extracts.

The second document, *Guidance for the Retail Labeling of Dietary Supplements Containing Soft or Powdered Botanical Extracts*, offers standards for the labeling of consumer goods containing these herbal ingredients. When adopted broadly, the AHPA hopes conformity to the established norms will lead to greater communication with the end users of herbal products and provide information that will assist in product differentiation.

Finally, a "white paper" entitled *Use of Marker Compounds in Manufacturing and Labeling Botanically Derived Dietary Supplements* defines and discusses several of the constituents that naturally occur in herbs and that are "selected for special attention by a researcher or manufacturer." The largest part of this document is devoted to evaluating the benefits and pitfalls of identifying these compounds in research, manufacturing, and marketing.

The three documents are available from AHPA, e-mail: ahpa@ahpa.org and website: www.ahpa.org.

Quality Assurance

Quality control

One of the major concerns of government authorities of producing countries and promoters of the kava industry is the need to ensure the marketing of only high quality product. At present there are no quality control or management procedures in place. Thus, in recognition of this need, some of the relevant countries have set up bodies to coordinate all aspects of the kava industry. In Fiji, it is called the Fiji National Kava Council. In 1999, a regional organization, called the Pacific Island Kava Council, had its inaugural meeting in Vanuatu with participants from Fiji, Samoa, Tonga, Vanuatu, the Federated States of Micronesia, Hawai'i, and Wallis and Futuna. The major recommendation of the group called for the promotion and development of kava through research, new and improved methods of processing, quality assurance and setting of guidelines for standardized products sold as genuine kava, and formulation of international marketing strategies. These countries also felt that since kava is indigenous to that region of the world and is an essential item for their economy, special protection should be sought for and granted to the industry by the international community.

In recognition of the economic importance of kava to the island nations and to ensure the quality of the marketed item, the Secretariat of the Pacific Community (SPC) funded the Institute of Applied Sciences of the University of the South Pacific, the main campus of which is in Suva, Fiji, to develop quality specifications for kava. The draft quality specifications have now been formulated and form part of a manual entitled, "*Pacific Kava: A Producer's Guide*," which is being prepared for publication by SPC. In the draft manual, the following quality specifications are proposed.

Description

The kava will be the roots, rootstock, basal stems or scrapings, which will be clean, and substantially free of dirt, soil, and other contaminants. It will be prepared using good manufacturing practice, and will not contain vegetable matter derived from other plant species, insect fragments, or any other extraneous matter. In addition, it will have the following properties.

COLOR

Kava will have the characteristic light brown/grey color.

AROMA

Kava will have the characteristic aroma of the product. It should be devoid of extraneous aromas indicating contamination with other plant material, solvents, or other volatile matter.

FLAVOR

In the event of dispute, kava samples will be subject to a taste panel assessment using the triangular taste test. There will be at least 20 panelists and the results will be subjected to statistical analysis. Samples with statistically significant differences from test samples will be treated as contaminated.

DIRT (FILTH)

Heavy dirt will not exceed 0.65% on a dry weight basis. Kava with heavy dirt between 0.63 and 0.70% will be considered to be second grade. Samples with heavy dirt exceeding 0.70% will need to be rewashed and redried.

MOISTURE

The moisture content will not exceed 12.54% when dried to constant weight at 105 °C. Kava with moisture content between 12.54 and 12.88% will be considered second grade. Samples with moisture content in excess of 12.88% will need to be redried.

ASH

The ash content will not exceed 5.36% when organic matter is removed at 440 °C. Kava giving ash between 5.36 and 5.93% will be considered to be second grade. Samples with ash content in excess of 5.93% will need to be washed and redried.

KAVALACTONES

The quality specification for kavalactone content is still under development and is very difficult to specify because of the great variability among the different cultivars.

However, if large consignments are involved, the buyer and seller should test for the kavalactone content, which can then form the basis for price negotiations.

Adulterants

The adulteration of powdered kava in the Fijian market was first reported by Duve and Prasad (1981), but it was common knowledge even before this. Although all adulterants have not been scientifically identified, there are a number of probable candidates. In Fiji, sawdust, flour, and the dregs from the extraction of sugarcane, which are plentiful during the cane harvesting season have all been implicated. The possible inclusion of plant parts of related species of *Piper* or *Macropiper* in the genuine kava product has also been suggested. The fibrous residue from kava extractions (called *makas* in the Bislama language in Vanuatu) is probably a more likely suspect (Lebot *et al.*, 1997). After the preparation of the beverage, the kava residue is relatively rich in fiber, but very deficient in kavalactones. Such adulteration with kava residue could explain variations in the strength of kava powders sold on the Fijian market, although this variation may also be a reflection of cultivars with different chemotypes. Experienced consumers are well aware of adulteration in powdered kava and thus often prefer to buy the kavastock to be privately powdered by hand.

Quality markers of kava

Since the kavalactones are the main psychoactive ingredients for which kava is produced, they provide a useful starting point for quality control. The use of TLC and spectrophotometry (Young *et al.*, 1966; Csupor, 1970) and GLC (Achenbach *et al.*, 1971; Duve and Prasad, 1981; Smith, 1983; Duffield *et al.*, 1989) provided reliable methods for determining the kavalactone composition and content in the kava plant. But they proved to be cumbersome and time-consuming and would obviously be unfeasible for regular quality control purposes. Advances in normal HPLC (Gracza and Ruff, 1980; Smith *et al.*, 1984) and reverse phase HPLC (Boonen *et al.*, 1997; Shao *et al.*, 1998; Ganzera and Khan, 1999) specifically for kavalactones, have made it possible to do both qualitative and quantitative analyses with relative ease and great accuracy.

Typical HPLC methods

In early 1998, the Institute for Nutraceutical Advancement (INA) with the support of 30 sponsoring companies, launched the INA Methods Validation Program (INA MVP), an international project designed to select, validate, and publish scientific methods for use in analyzing raw botanical materials. At the time of writing, the INA website (*www.nsfina.org*) provides the methods for the following products: kavalactones in *Piper methysticum*, flavonol glycosides and terpenoids in ginkgo (*Ginkgo biloba*), ginsenosides in Asian ginseng (*Panax ginseng*) and American ginseng (*Panax quinquefolius*), eleutherosides in Siberian ginseng (*Eleutherococcus senticosus*), hypericin, pseudohypericin, and hyperforin in St John's wort (*Hypericum perforatum*), total polyphenols in *Echinacea*, allicin in garlic (*Allium sativum*), total catechins and gallic acid in green tea (*Camellia sinensis*), gingerols and shogaols in ginger (*Zingiber officinale*), silymarins in milk thistle (*Silybum marianum*), triterpene glycosides in black cohosh (*Cimicifuga racemosa*), and isoflavone glucosides and aglycones in soy and powdered soy extract, all by HPLC; fatty acids and sterols in saw palmetto (*Serenoa repens*) by gas chromatography, and anthocyanin content in bilberry (*Vaccinium myrtillus*) by pH-differential spectrophotometry.

The INA MVP procedure for kavalactones was modified from Shao *et al.* (1998). This method is suitable for the six major kavalactones in either crude plant material or soft extracts. Briefly, the sample is extracted by sonication at room temperature in a methanol:water (70:30 v/v) mixture for crude plant material for 60 minutes or in methanol for soft extract or paste for 10 minutes or until dissolved. Standard solutions of the six kavalactones are prepared by dissolving in methanol by sonication. The chromatographic conditions are: YMCbasic C8 column, 5 μM particle size, 250×4.6 mm, or equivalent, isocratic 0.1% phosphoric acid:isopropyl alcohol: acetonitrile (64:16:20 v/v) mobile phase, 1.0 ml/min flow rate, injection volume 5 μl, detection wavelength 220 nm, and running time 40 minutes. Kavain, dihydrokavain, methysticin, dihydromethysticin, yangonin, and desmethoxyyangonin comprise the kavalactone standards.

In the Ganzera and Khan (1999) method, crude plant material was extracted in methanol by sonication and filtered through a 0.45 μM membrane filter. The kavalactone standards were dissolved in acetone. The column was a Luna C8, 100×4.6 mm, 3 μM particle size (from Phenomenex, Torrance, California). The mobile phase was water:acetonitrile: reagent alcohol (65:20:15 v/v). Chromatographic conditions were: flow rate 0.5 ml/min, detection wavelength 246 nm, injection volume 5 μl, and running time 45 minutes.

Marketing and Economics

Until about 20–30 years ago, the main demand for kava was for the drinking market in the South Pacific and to a lesser extent by immigrants from this area to North America, Europe, Australia, and New Zealand. Since the renaissance of herbal medicine use in the West, the interest in kava by the pharmaceutical and nutraceutical industry and hence its demand and commercial value dramatically increased. With the gaining of political independence and the acquisition of self-determination by most of the island countries during this same time period, local kava consumption has increased, even where it previously was only used for ritualistic and medicinal purposes. This upward trend has also in part been due to the policy of some of the governments of promoting kava as a traditional and socially acceptable alternative to alcohol. As a result the importance of kava as an agricultural product became on par with copra, ginger, bananas, etc., and in Fiji only sugar surpassed its production. However, the recent reports on kava-associated liver toxicity have severely curtailed the volume of kava exports from the producing countries. The economic impact of the reported liver toxicity is discussed later in this chapter.

Kava has many advantages as a cash crop. Since it has been an indigenous crop for many generations, the farmers are familiar with production techniques and the government authorities do not have to struggle to increase its production. Ample supplies of the planting material are available, both small- and large-scale production are feasible, and the market prices are relatively stable. It can be easily intercropped with many other crops, while it is possible to plant it as a monocrop as well. Kava is also relatively resistant to hurricane damage which is always possible in the South Pacific. From an economic perspective, it has a higher cash return per work day compared to its normal competitors, such as coconuts, cocoa, coffee, garlic, ginger, black pepper, and vanilla. For instance, Lebot *et al.* (1997) have estimated the following comparative cash crop income in Vanuatu in 1985 as (calculated by dividing net income per hectare by the number of work days required over the full crop cycle, in US$): kava 25.15, vanilla 17.71, cardamom 11.37, garlic 10.83, pepper 9.03, cocoa 8.96, coffee 8.00, ginger 6.88, and copra 5.00. A similar comparison for Fiji shows a larger gross economic return for kava compared to other selected crops, namely (Fijian$/person/day), kava 75–85, mango 38–42, taro 14–16, ginger 11–20, vanilla 7–10, sugarcane 6–9, copra 3–5, and bulk cocoa 4–5 (Kumar *et al.*, 1998).

Trading systems and networks

Since kava is a perishable item, it needs to be transported directly from the growers on the outer islands or remote areas on the larger islands to the urban centers. Inter-island ships which transport other produce, like copra, cocoa, coffee, etc., also ferry the dried kava. Often there is a middleman on the island or farm area in the larger islands to coordinate the collection from the farmers, or alternatively they may transport the kava directly to the middleman in town (Figure 3.3). However, there are a number of difficulties in maintaining a steady supply of kava for both the drinking and pharma-ceutical markets. Kava has been largely grown in a vast area over which relatively small family-owned plots of the crop are scattered. This means the local middleman has to travel large distances to pick up small quantities of the produce, thereby increasing the operational costs. If the grower makes the delivery, this also involves traveling long distances and additionally requires using expensive commercial transportation, which act as disincentives for the grower to make his own delivery.

The irregularity in supply is also closely linked to the subsistence mentality of the community, so that many farmers simply leave the crop in the ground and only harvest it when there is pressing financial need. So there may be a glut of kava at Christmas time after long periods of insufficient or erratic supply during rest of the year. Another feature of the grower to processor marketing of kava is the wide variation in type and

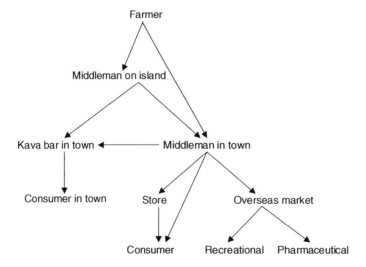

Figure 3.3 Marketing channels for kava in the major producing countries. Adapted from *Kava, the Pacific Elixir* by V. Lebot, M. Merlin, and L. Lindstrom, 2nd edition, 1997, Figure 6.3, and produced with permission from the publisher, Yale University Press.

quality of what the processor receives. Some processors prefer the growers to simply harvest the crop, attempt no in-field processing at all, but deliver or sell it directly to them, as they can then control the quality of the kava. This means the processors are in charge of the full range of tasks of washing, chipping and peeling, sorting, drying, pulverizing, sieving, and packing. However, this is advisable only if the freshly harvested crops are delivered to the processing plants within a very short time – no more than a couple of day – or deterioration rapidly sets in.

Economic role as a cash crop

Until about 1995–96, the major demand for kava was for local consumption in the South Pacific countries, with a small quantity being exported to pharmaceutical concerns in Europe and Pacific Island emigrants in Western countries. Production, which had been increasing gradually up to this time, rose dramatically, then settled at a lower plateau for the next few years (Table 3.1). For instance, kava export from Fiji was (in US currency) 1.53×10^6 in 1997, 15.76×10^6 in 1998, then decreased to about 2.5×10^6 during 1999–2001. A similar trend can be seen for Vanuatu (Table 3.1).

In the past few years, the destination for the majority of kava export from Fiji and Vanuatu, the two major producers, has been six different countries (see Figure 3.4; Nawalowalo, 2002). For 2001, the most recent year for which official data are available from Fiji, the kava export values (in US currency) to these countries were as follows: Germany, $866,000; USA, $615,500; Spain, $295,000; New Zealand, $243,000; Australia, $143,500; and Saudi Arabia, $113,900, which together comprised about 93% of the total kava export from Fiji. Other data relating to production and local consumption in Fiji are shown in Table 3.1.

Comparable data from Vanuatu are less readily available. However, it has been estimated that the number of kava plants in cultivation rose from about 1.289 million in 1983 to 3.694 million in 1994 and 6.066 million in 1999. In the same years, the kava planting

Table 3.1 Production and marketing data for kava in Fiji and Vanuatu, 1997–2002

	1997	1998	1999	2000	2001	2002*
Planting area (ha)						
Fiji	1892	3115	1785	1542	1658	na
Production (000 kg)						
Fiji	3363	3254	3028	2925	5244	na
Export[§] volume (000 kg)						
Fiji	369	1376	301	373	418	138
Vanuatu	105	749	334	555	935	438
Export[§] value (000 USD)						
Fiji	1530	15,763	2688	2445	2440	818
Vanuatu	729	6342	2707	3414	3593	1257
LC[¶] volume (000 kg)						
Fiji	3852	1923	2780	2756	5020	na

Sources: King (2002) and Nawalowalo (2002).

Notes
ha – in hectares; na – not available.
* projections for 2002 based on data from January to September 2002.
§ to other than the major kava-producing countries.
¶ LC – local consumption; includes material imported from other major kava-producing countries.

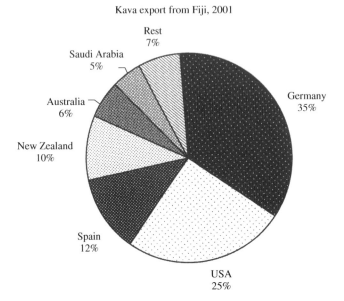

Figure 3.4 Destinations of kava for pharmaceutical and recreational purposes exported from Fiji during 2001. Data provided by Fiji National Kava Council.

areas were 1,290, 2,462, and 3,033 ha, respectively (King, 2002). The dramatic increase during the period between 1983 and 1999 in the number of kava plants in cultivation on the various islands of Vanuatu is indicated in Figure 3.5. During most of the 1990s, the local market in green or fresh kava, the major form for use in Vanuatu, was about 6.1×10^6 kg, equivalent to 1.22×10^6 kg of dried kava, and was worth roughly US$570,000. This figure does not include kava produced and used by farmers without it entering the local commercial market. According to information supplied by Patricia Siméoni (personal communication, December 2002), 12.73×10^6 kg of fresh kava was used in this manner in the year 2000. At the same time the domestic market, accounted for 7.64×10^6 kg, and 2.55×10^6 kg were exported, all as green kava, giving a total production figure for the year of about 22.9×10^6 kg.

The ban or suspension of kava sales in some countries and health advisories in others in 2001 has had a dramatic impact on kava demand from pharmaceutical companies. At the time of writing, no final production or export data are available for 2002. However, the Bureau of Statistics of the Fiji and Vanuatu Governments have projected that, based on the data reported in the first nine months of the year, kava exports from these two countries will be about 60–67% less in 2002 than in the previous three years (Table 3.1). This turn of events has had a devastating effect on many small farmers who had switched from other crops to kava production on encouragement from their governments and in anticipation of continued high demand. Since a resolution of the concern linking kava with liver toxicity may take some years and still leave a stigma on the herb even if found not to be causally responsible for the toxicity, the adverse impact on the industry and the livelihood of the affected farmers and their communities will undoubtedly be severe and prolonged.

Nombre de kavas par îles en 1983 et en 1999

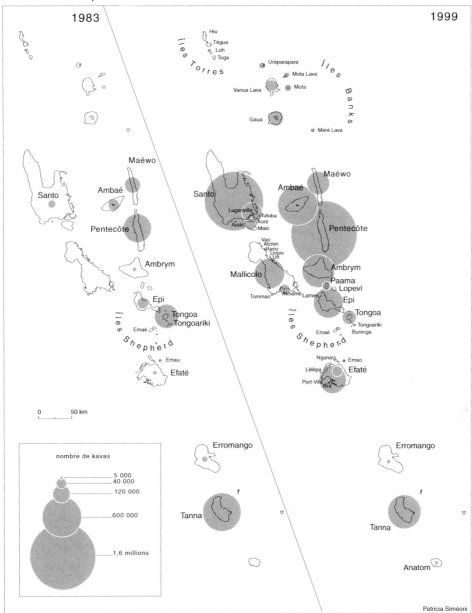

Figure 3.5 The marked increase in kava production in Vanuatu between 1983 and 1999 indicated by the number of plants under cultivation on the various islands of the group. Reproduced with permission of Dr Patricia Siméoni from her Ph.D. dissertation, *"Buveurs de Kava: Genèse et Variabilité Géographique des Notions de Qualité,"* University of Paris, Sorbonne, 2003.

While the reports of liver toxicity have raised some concerns with recreational users of kava, they have not had a similar downturn on usage by this group as in the pharmaceutical market. Consequently, the consumption locally in the South Pacific and by Pacific emigrants in other countries has not been drastically affected, to the great relief of the growers and producers. However, the research and development efforts that were in progress in order to increase production and product quality have to some extent been put on hold while the question of liver toxicity is being resolved.

References

Achenbach, H., Karl, W. and Smith, S. (1971) Inhaltsstoffe des Rauschpfeffers. IV. Zur gaschromatographischen Trennung der Kawa-Lactone − (+)-5,6,7,8-Tetrahydro-yangonin, ein neues Kawa-Lacton aus Rauschpfeffer. *Chemische Berichte*, **104**, 2688–2693.

Bhat, S.R., Chandel, K.P.S. and Malik, S.K. (1995) Plant regeneration from various explants of cultivated *Piper* species. *Plant Cell Reports*, **14**, 398–402.

Boonen, G., Beck, M.A. and Haberlein, H. (1997) Contribution to the quantitative and enantio-selective determination of kavapyrones by high performance liquid chromatography on ChiraSpher NT material. *Journal of Chromatography B*, **703**, 240–244.

Brown, J.F. (1989) *Kava and Kava Diseases in the South Pacific*, Paper No. 24, ACIAR, Canberra, Australia.

Brown, J.F. and Minchinton, E.J. (1989) Kava and kava diseases in the South Pacific: an overview and summary. In Brown, J.F. (ed.), *Kava and Kava Diseases in the South Pacific*, Paper No. 24, ACIAR, Canberra, Australia.

Butler, L.D. (1973) *Yaqona wilt investigation*, Annual Research Report for 1972. Department of Agriculture, Suva, Fiji, pp. 132–133.

Butler, L.D. (1974) *Common Economic Plant Diseases in Fiji*, Ministry of Agriculture, Fisheries, and Forests, Fiji, 37pp.

Csupor, L. (1970) Die quantitative Bestimmung der Kawa-Laktone in *Piper methysticum* (Forster). Bestimmungsmethoden mit den Reinsubstanzen Kawain, Methysticin und Yangonin. *Archiv der Pharmazie*, **303**(3), 193–200.

Davis, R.I. and Brown, J.F. (1999) *Kava (Piper methysticum) in the South Pacific*, ACIAR Technical Reports 46, ACIAR, Canberra, Australia.

Davis, R.I., Brown, J.F. and Pone, S.P. (1996) Causal relationship between cucumber mosaic cucumvirus and kava dieback in the South Pacific. *Plant Disease*, **80**, 194–198.

Duffield, A., Jamieson, D., Lidgard, R., Duffield, P. and Bourne, D. (1989) Identification of some human urinary metabolites of the intoxicating beverage kava. *Journal of Chromatography*, **475**, 273–282.

Duve, R.N. and Prasad, J. (1981) Quality evaluation of yaqona (*Piper methysticum*) in Fiji. *Fiji Agriculture Journal*, **43**, 1–8.

Fakalata, O. (1981) Weevil pest on kava stems in Vava'u (Tonga). *Alafua Agricultural Bulletin*, **6**, 38–39.

Fakalata, O. and Langi, T. (1983) *Kava project profiles*, Unpublished internal report of the German-Tongan Plant Protection Project, pp. 1–9.

Fitchet, M. (1990) Establishment of *Piper nigrum in vitro*. *Acta Horticulture*, **275**, 285–291.

Ganzera, M. and Khan, I. (1999) Analytical techniques for the determination of lactones in *Piper methysticum* Forst. *Chromatographia*, **50**, 649–653.

Gerlach, W.W.P. (1988) *Plant Diseases of Western Samoa*, Samoa-German Crop Protection Project, Apia, Western Samoa, 215pp.

Gracza, L. and Ruff, P. (1980) Einfache Methode zur Trennung und quantitativen Bestimmung von Kawa-Laktonen durch Hochleistungs-Flussigkeits-Chromatographie. *Journal of Chromatograhy*, 193, 486–490.

Heinlein, M., Kumar, J., Nambiar, V., Kaitetara, T. and Kashyap, D.M. (1984) *Yaqona Pests and Diseases Wilt and Stem Rot Control in Yaqona*, Annual Research Report for 1983, Department of Agriculture, Suva, Fiji, pp. 51–52.

King, F. (2002) Addressing the socio-economic dimension of the current kava problem. *Pacific Kava Research Symposium*. November 6–7, 2002, Suva, Fiji.

Kumar, J., Singh, D.S., Kaitetara, T., Nambiar, V. and Kashyap, D.M. (1985) *Yaqona: Pests and Diseases. Yaqona Disease Complex*, Annual Research Report for 1985, Department of Agriculture, Suva, Fiji, 44pp.

Kumar, S., Kaitetera, T. and Mudaliar, T. (1998) *Opportunities for Production of Yaqona in Fiji for Export. Situation Analysis No. 1*, Fiji Ministry of Agriculture, Forestry, and Fisheries, and Crop Evaluation Project, AusAID, Suva.

Lebot, V., Merlin, M. and Lindstrom, L. (1997) *Kava, the Pacific Elixir*, Healing Arts Press, Rochester, Vermont.

MAFF (2001) Fiji Ministry of Agriculture, Forestry, and Fisheries, Suva, Annual Report for 2000.

Nawalowalo, J. (2002) Historical significance of kava in Fiji and its commercial value in the international markets. *Pacific Kava Research Symposium*. November 6–7, 2002, Suva, Fiji.

Orton Williams, K.J. (1980) *Plant Parasitic Nematodes of the South Pacific*, Technical Report Volume 8, Commonwealth Institute of Helminthology, St. Albans, Australia, 192pp.

Pares, R.D., Gillings, M.R., Davis, R.I. and Brown, J.F. (1992) Cucumber mosaic cucumvirus associated with kava plants showing symptoms of dieback disease in Fiji and Tonga. *Australasian Plant Pathology*, 21, 169–171.

Parham, B.E.V. (1935) Wilt disease of "yaqona". *Fiji Agricultural Journal*, 8, 2–8.

Shao, Y., He, K., Zheng, B. and Zheng, Q. (1998) Reversed phase high performance liquid chromatographic method for quantitative analysis of the six major kavalactones in *Piper methysticum*. *Journal of Chromatography A*, 825, 1–18.

Singh, P. and Nambiar, V. (1988) *Yaqona: Control of Yaqona Wilt Disease*, Annual Report for 1987, Research Division, Fiji Department of Agriculture, Suva.

Smith, R.M. (1983) Kavalactones on *Piper methysticum* from Fiji. *Phytochemistry*, 22(4), 1055–1056.

Smith, R.M., Thakrar, H., Arowolo, T.A. and Shafi, A.A. (1984) High performance liquid chromatography of kava lactones from *Piper methysticum*. *Journal of Chromatography*, 283, 303–308.

Taylor, D.M. and Taufa, L. (1998) Decontamination of kava (*Piper methysticum*) for *in vitro* propagation. *Acta Horticulture*, 461, 267–274.

Young, R.L., Hylin, J.W., Plucknett, D.L., Kawano, Y. and Nakayama, R.T. (1966) Analysis for kawa pyrones in extracts of *Piper methysticum*. *Phytochemistry*, 5(4), 795–798.

4 Botany and Ethnobotany of Kava

Yadhu N. Singh

Introduction

Like most traditional Pacific crops, kava is propagated vegetatively by stem cuttings. Its cultivars are all cloned, so that cloning of a single individual results in a genetically identical progeny. The point of origin, dispersal, and discontinuous distribution of kava, its link to the history of human migration, and whether it shares the main migratory routes of other Pacific crops into and across Oceania remains unresolved. The origin of kava has been described variously as "problematical" (Yuncker, 1959); "uncertain" (Smith, 1981); as a native of eastern Indonesia or Papua New Guinea (Newell, 1947; Barrau, 1965); in south China (Handy, 1927); in southern India (Williamson, 1939); or in western Melanesia (Brunton, 1989), in particular, in Vanuatu (Lebot *et al.*, 1997). Previously, theories on domestication of kava were largely based on the pattern of its geographic distribution and comparative linguistic analysis of vernacular names. Recent morphological and genetic research perhaps provide a more convincing picture of kava's taxonomic relations, as well as its origins and distribution throughout the Pacific (Lebot *et al.*, 1997).

This chapter discusses the plant's past and present geographic distribution, taxonomic relations and morphology, and the theories on the origins of kava based on morphological, genetic, and geographical evidence, and linguistic analysis of vernacular names.

Geography of Distribution

Although often identified with western Polynesia, kava was in the past found in nearly all Pacific islands. Ethnographic accounts reveal that kava died out in many of the localities and islands through neglect, devastation by wild animals like pigs, or competition from natural vegetation, weeds, and climbing vines. Both dispersal and continued survival of the plant depend on human attention, without which it often declines and disappears from the environment within a few decades. However, as a relic of cultivation, kava can thrive, albeit for limited periods of time, in well-protected rain forests where vegetative propagation occurs from living stems falling to the ground. The decline or disappearance of kava usage in many island communities usually arose from the condemnation and often ban by Christian missionaries because of its association with so-called non-Christian practices, in an effort by colonizers to gain political control by lessening the pre-eminent position of the chiefs and elders with whom kava usage was closely associated, and the disapproval by Western medical personnel who considered the chewing method of kava preparation to be unhygienic (Singh, 1992).

Examination of collected specimens in 19 of the largest herbaria in the world (Lebot and Lévesque, 1989), coupled with various field trips (Lebot, 1991) and bibliographic research, has resulted in the identification of the past and present areas of distribution of kava in the Pacific. Presently it is cultivated most prominently in Fiji, Tonga, (American and Western) Samoa, Vanuatu, Wallis and Futuna, Pohnpei (Ponape), and some areas of Papua New Guinea. In the past it was found in Tahiti (in the Society Islands), Cook Islands, the Marquesas, Hawai'i (although it is once again being cultivated there), Niue, Santa Cruz, and Kosrae (previously Kusaie). Kava has not been recorded from New Caledonia, Solomons (except for some contradictory reports), Nauru, Tuvalu, Guam, Palau, Truk, Norfolk, and Rapa (Figure 1.3). The situation in a few cases is uncertain, e.g. Tokelau, as conflicting claims of previous presence or complete absence are found in the literature (Lebot *et al.*, 1997). The absence of kava from the smaller flat coral atolls is understandable as the plant cannot grow there because of unsuitable ecological conditions.

Geographic origin and dispersal

The origins of kava and its methods of dispersal across Oceania are not known. Kava usage itself is much older than any documented history of this part of the world and oral traditions do not seem to have brought forward relevant, reliable, or consistent accounts. It should be noted that at first contact with Europeans none of the island communities had an alphabet, and therefore a written language of their own. Furthermore, the journal entries that are available are very much from the Eurocentric point of view, especially of the explorers, travelers, and Christian missionaries. However, a consideration of some of these accounts provides an insight not available from other sources.

According to Rivers (1914), the kava custom was related to, or evolved out of, an earlier established practice of betel nut chewing. In fact, Rivers has suggested the presence of two distinct cultural traditions in Oceania: the betel nut culture and the kava culture. Betel nut chewing involves three separate ingredients – crushed nut of the areca palm (*Areca catechu* L.), leaves of *Piper betle* L., and slaked lime, while kava requires only one ingredient. Rivers believes that partly because of this, kava drinking succeeded betel nut chewing as migrants were unable to acquire all the necessary components for the earlier habit. Rivers also thinks that kava arose in part as a result of the needs encountered by the immigrants under alien conditions and who found the kava root more satisfying as a drug than the betel nut. This latter suggestion is queried by Williamson (1939) on two counts. First, both the betel nut and the kava plant grow in the same areas of New Guinea and Samoa, and yet, in New Guinea, kava is of minor importance, whereas in Samoa betel nut chewing is virtually unknown. Second, the fact that kava is in fact far less potent as a drug than the betel nut also somewhat discredits the reason given by Rivers for the immigrants' preference for kava over the betel nut.

Churchill (1916) also proposes the presence of two cultures based on the distribution of kava and betel in Oceania. He suggests that these two cultures belonged to two migrant peoples whom he called "the kava people" and "the betel people." The kava people settled in southern Melanesia, Fiji, and Polynesia while the betel people did not extend in the southeasterly movement beyond the Solomons and Santa Cruz Islands. However, certain elements of the culture of the betel people may have carried directly or indirectly to southern Melanesia, Fiji, and Polynesia, although it appears to be minimal and any that does exist is probably of recent origin.

According to Newell (1947), the origin of the kava plant appears to have been in the New Guinea–Indonesia area or further north. This is a little west of a more botanically based conclusion reached by Lebot (discussed later in this chapter) that kava most likely originated in Vanuatu and its neighboring islands. Newell proposes three different ways in which the plant could have been spread to Tonga and eastern Pacific by, namely: (a) the islands having been attached to a main land mass on which kava evolved and developed; (b) drifting or being otherwise transported from island to island; and (c) being transported in canoes by man.

The first of these proposals may be discounted, as most of the islands of Oceania are of comparatively recent geological origin and consist of coral limestones or volcanic cones. The possibility that the plant or its root drifted to the various islands on which it is now found seems equally remote because of the great distances and the large number of islands involved. Thus, without completely discounting the first two possibilities, Newell concludes that the kava root or plant was brought by early Polynesian explorers in much the same way as they brought other plants in their canoes.

Newell's contention is that kava did not spread eastward from a center of origin in the New Guinea-Indonesia area through the Solomons and nearby territories. Rather, it was transported through the Caroline and the Marshall Islands in Micronesia to Hawai'i on the one hand or, alternatively, through Tuvalu to eastern Polynesia. The obvious route for the spread of kava to central and eastern Polynesia is through the Solomons. He argues that if the hypothesis is accepted, it is difficult to explain why the kava custom became the center of an important ritual in Fiji, Tonga, and Samoa but has been of little importance – indeed virtually non-existent – in most of the Solomons through which the practice should have been transported.

The second hypothesis places the origins of the kava custom on the Asian subcontinent. In his works on the cultural origins of Polynesians, Handy (1927) proposes that different cultures of the Polynesian area are the product of evolution within Polynesia itself. That is, of a single culture which the original Polynesians brought with them. He compares various cultural traits of Polynesians with those found in Southern China and connects the drinking of kava in Polynesia with the ancient Chinese tea ceremony.

Williamson (1939), on the other hand, thinks that the Polynesians might have originated slightly further west, in the southern parts of India. In a detailed account, he argues that the kava ceremony might equally well be compared with the ceremonials, rituals, and beliefs connected with the drinking of *soma* in the ancient Vedic religion, a ceremony to which it bears considerable resemblance. He discusses many points of similarity between the kava ceremony and the Vedic ritual. The fixed number of priests who participated in the *soma* ritual is reminiscent of the formalized kava ring, in which each person had a clearly defined place and function. In particular, the Vedic prohibition against a younger brother offering a sacrifice before his older brother, has a remarkable parallel in the rule governing the precedence of brothers in the kava ring. Again the honoring and invoking of deities, together with the pouring out of libations of the beverage were features of both cults. Furthermore, there was, as with kava, a ritualistic manner of preparation of the beverage by beating – in the earliest times with stones; later with mortar and pestle – and by straining the liquid into wooden vats. The last two features present a striking parallel to the preliminary breaking up of kava roots with stones, the squeezing of kava juice and its reception in the wooden kava bowl (Williamson, 1939).

Following dispersal and establishment in the different island groups, kava developed its role in the lives of the inhabitants. In Hawai'i, the people placed great importance on kava drinking as late as the end of the nineteenth century (Emerson, 1903). Titcomb (1948) states that the kava custom was highly esteemed in Hawai'i because it was a sacred drink of great significance in many phases of Hawaiian life. Outside of water and coconut milk, no other drink was known. Its effect was to relax the mind and body and it was used by farmers and fishermen alike for this purpose. Medical *kahunas* (priests or learned men) had many uses for it. It was customary for chiefs to drink it before meals, commoners also if it was obtainable. It was essential on occasions of hospitality and feasting and was the drink of leisure of the chiefs. However, the sale and use of kava rapidly declined from the beginning of the twentieth century. Titcomb (1948) noted that in 1903, no Hawaiian went home from the Saturday market without an 'awa' root tied to his saddle. By 1948, the practice had largely disappeared, although the plant continued to grow in the wild. In the last 10–15 years serious consideration has been given to the exploitation of kava as a commercial crop on some of the land previously engaged in sugar cane production.

Kava usage has been of major importance in Vanuatu, where it is drunk socially, but not ceremonially, and where the plant is recognized as a remedy for many important ailments. At present, kava bars and clubs, called *nakamals* in the local language (*Bislama*), are popular centers for social gathering of urban men throughout Vanuatu. The urban nakamals have retained some of the character and functions of traditional island nakamals – the houses or forest clearings in which men gather to drink kava and socialize. The resurgence of kava drinking which was noted on the Vanuatu island of Tanna in the early 1940s may be related to the ritual of the John Frum cargo cult, which arose partly as a repudiation of the teachings of the Christian missionaries (Guiart, 1956). Carlton Gadjusek (the Nobel Laureate who is credited with identifying *kuru*, the slow developing brain disorder of New Guinea highlanders) spent several weeks on another island of this group, Tongariki. He found that the prevailing kava drinking practice there was more like that of the early John Frum movement on Tanna in its lack of formality and restraints (Gadjusek, 1979).

In historic times, the most important centers of kava usage probably were Fiji, Samoa, and Tonga. In these countries it was consumed not merely as a beverage but had become the focus of an elaborate system of social ceremonials and rituals and also had certain healing and magico-religious aspects. In the last few decades of the twentieth century kava began to regain some of its earlier importance. This may be closely linked to the gaining of political independence and the subsequent reassertion of ethnic values, customs, and priorities which had been suppressed or discouraged during the colonial era lasting a century or more.

The occurrence of kava in the Solomons has been contentious. According to Rivers (1914), kava was drunk in the Solomon islands of Vanikoro and Utupua, whereas Codrington (1891) and Thomson (1908) claimed it to be unknown in the Santa Cruz Islands. Fox (1924) related that men drank kava at burial ceremonies but not on other occasions. The only island in the Solomons group reported to have contemporary knowledge of kava and its uses is Choiseul where some islanders claim it is used medicinally. Rennell Island at the bottom end of the archipelago does not have *P. methysticum* but has a coconut drink which curiously is called *kava kava ngangi* (Holmes, 1979).

Kava was, during the nineteenth century, grown on all islands of the Cooks group but the infusion which was usually prepared from the root of the plant did not have the same ceremonial significance as it did in western Polynesia (Hiroa, 1944). However, it is now virtually impossible to locate the plant on any of these islands and the practices relating to it seem to have completely disappeared.

It is asserted by Turner (1861) and Hood (1862) that kava was not drunk in Niue. Percy Smith (1920) states that the Niue people did not make or use the drink and drew attention to the difference in this respect between them and the Samoans and Tongans with whom they are closely connected, suggesting that the reason for this may have been the scarcity of the plant. Thomson (1902) found that kava was not used as a beverage by the Niueans but was used for inspiration by their priests.

Scarcity is the reason sometimes given for the fact that in Tahiti kava drinking was only indulged in by the chiefs (Parkinson, 1784; Wilson, 1799). Although the kava root was scarce and little used in Tahiti, there were large plantations of it in the other Society Islands (Forster, 1777). This suggests that it was probably a lack of desire rather than of supply which limited kava drinking by the natives of Tahiti, as they could presumably have obtained supplies from the other nearby islands if they so desired. Cultivation of kava in Tahiti declined sharply after the arrival of missionaries, so that after 1830 "it was no longer possible to find a single specimen of the plant and many Tahitians no longer even knew it by name" (Lewin, 1924). Nevertheless, Cuzent (1857) was able to collect over a dozen different kava cultivars between 1854 and 1857 on Tahiti.

On Wallis Island (called Uvea in Polynesian), the position of the kava ceremony was as highly esteemed as anywhere else in the Pacific (Mangeret, 1884). All official decisions and promulgations concerning the community's administration, such as promotions, official takings of possessions, proclaiming of laws and codes of conduct, were made at such ceremonies. The kava root was often used in reconciling with enemies or in preserving the goodwill of kings and chiefs. Indeed, guilty persons often owed their pardon and sometimes even their lives to it. In the neighbouring island of Futuna, as elsewhere in the South Pacific, kava was used to express friendship and to allay fear. Mangeret (1884) notes that once, on the arrival of a French ship, the native people, fearing vengeance for the murder of a missionary a few months earlier, presented the captain with an enormous kava root.

Thomson (1889) states that kava was not grown, nor was the drink known on Easter Island. Perhaps the climatic conditions were not favorable. This, however, cannot explain why kava was not cultivated on Rapa where the climate was favorable (Métraux, 1940). Kava has also been found in Tuvalu (formerly called the Ellice Islands), the Caroline Islands where it occurs only on Pohnpei and where it is called *sakau*, and on Kosrae (Krieger, 1943). In Pohnpei, the cultural elements associated with kava drinking indicate a closer relationship with Vanuatu than with Polynesia (Brunton, 1989) and provide strong evidence that kava was introduced to Micronesia from Melanesia. Kava also occurs in some of the "Polynesian outliers" (i.e., islands which lie in Melanesia but whose people are Polynesian in origin), although information here is quite scanty or unreliable except in the case of Tikopia.

Tikopia is unquestionably the most famous of the Polynesian outliers, mainly because of the extensive work done there by the renowned British anthropologist Sir Raymond Firth. In Tikopia the use of kava differs radically from its use in other areas of the Western Pacific. Firth (1970) contends that "historically there is little doubt that kava rites of Tikopia belonged to the same general series as those of Tonga, Samoa, and Fiji and may well have been imported from that area." In Tikopia, kava was and still is very rarely drunk. Most of the liquid is poured away in libations and the remainder usually emptied out on the ground before the bowl is wiped clean.

The distribution of kava in Papua New Guinea and Irian Jaya or West Papua is very spotty. Although Brunton (1989) could not construct a definitive history of kava dispersal in this area, linguistic affinities for about 40 recorded names clearly indicate that contacts and exchanges took place among the kava-using localities. In the past, the area of greatest kava use in Papua New Guinea was the Admirality Islands, in particular, Baluan, Lou, Pam, and Fedarb. On Lou, the remaining plants were destroyed when the inhabitants were converted to Christianity in about 1970 (Lebot *et al.*, 1997). Kava is still found in isolated spots in the Admiralty Islands, but most residents now prefer to chew betel. On the mainland, kava has been cultivated along the northeastern coastal areas of Madang and Morobe provinces for local consumption or for sale. According to Miklouho-Maclay (1886), all indications are that it was introduced to the region a little before his arrival in 1872. The third kava-using region of relevance lies in the hinterland of Papua New Guinea and extends into West Papua, the Indonesian province which occupies the western part of the island. During his visits, Lebot discovered that only one cultivar was planted in an area of about 90,000 km^2. However, in both the hinterland and West Papua, kava is difficult to grow because of the unsuitable environmental and climatic conditions (Lebot *et al.*, 1997). As a result, the plants which never survive more than two years must be carefully tended and shaded. All of these attributes indicate that *P. methysticum* and its use are alien introductions to Papua New Guinea and West Papua, with its cultivation being restricted to the coastal areas and their hinterland.

The Australian aborigines had no contact with kava until the early 1980s when they learned about it from missionaries who came to their communities from Fiji, Tonga, and other kava-growing societies in the South Pacific (Cawte, 1985). At about the same time, Aboriginal leaders visiting Fiji and Polynesia were impressed with the kava ceremony and advocated kava use as an alcohol substitute for their own communities (Moyles, 1983). Soon thereafter kava was introduced from Fiji to Aboriginal communities in Northern Australia and rapidly became a drug of abuse (Cawte, 1985; Smiles, 1987), probably because of a lack of ceremonial or traditional restraints controlling its use. This situation would fall in the realm of the "law of alien poisons" (Schenk, 1956; Adrian, 1996) in much the same way as alcohol affected Native American (American Indian) populations after the arrival of Europeans several hundred years ago and cannabis did in North America and Europe beginning in the 1960s. Estimates of individual consumption have ranged as high as fifty times the amount habitually consumed in the Pacific Islands. An epidemic of kava abuse had become a serious social and health problem (Cawte, 1986; Mathews *et al.*, 1988) – so much so that the perceived gravity of the situation prompted statements like "kava turns people into zombies" (Northern Territory News, March 11, 1987), "the kava killer" (Sunday Territorian, March 15, 1987) and "it is important that everyone learns about it before it combines with diseases like AIDS to wipe out whole Aboriginal communities" (Northern Territory News, March 16, 1987). For a detailed account of the impact of kava in Australian Aboriginal populations, see Prescott and McCall (1988).

Traditional classification and etymology

It is often stated that the origin of *P. methysticum* is one of the major riddles of the ethnobotany of Oceania, which may be partly clarified by the study of the vernacular names of the plant. Its most well-known term *kava* and the variant *kawa*, are used for both the plant and the beverage prepared from it. Other variants include *kava-kava*, a term now becoming very popular in the pharmaceutical or nutraceutical industry of North America and *kawa-kawa*. Sometimes the initial *k* of the words is dropped, mainly in Polynesia, and they become *ava, awa, ava-ava* or *awa-awa*. Alternatively, they may become *'ava, 'awa, 'ava-ava* or *'awa-awa*. The Maoris, on migration to New Zealand, did not find the kava plant in their new environment, nor does it appear they took the plant with them; in any case the weather is probably too cold for kava to grow there. So they applied the names kawa and kawa-kawa to the related plant *P. excelsum* which was much used in religious ceremonies. However, it was not made into a beverage (Rivers, 1914). The term kava and its cognates have been used in Polynesia to designate various properties of food and drink. In Hawai'i, it means "bitter," "sour," "sharp," or "pungent." In the Marquesas it signifies "bitter," "sour" or "sharp." In Tahiti, the range is broad, including "bitter," "sour," "acrid," "salty," "sharp," and "pungent" (Churchill, 1916).

In Fiji, kava is known by a wholly different word, *yaqona*, which evidently has no affinity to the Polynesian term. In Fijian orthography, the letter *q* stands for the sound *ng* and hence *yaqona* is pronounced as *yangona*. Lester (1941) reports that the word *qona* was used on the northwest coast of the main Fijian island of Viti Levu to denote both "beverage" and "bitter." He suggests that this may indicate that it was to this part of Fiji that kava was first introduced and that local people supplied the name yaqona which is now used throughout the Fijian archipelago.

Compared to Polynesia, the linguistic situation in Melanesia, especially the western parts, displays a far more complex and diverse pattern of vernacular names for kava. The numerous names together with the procedures for cultivation and consumption are related to the large number of tribal groups and languages or dialects, and the greater opportunity for cultivation provided by suitable land and weather conditions. In addition, the longer history of kava use in Melanesia may be another important reason. Lebot and Cabalion (1988) list 35–40 different vernacular kava names, each from a different language area of the country. A strong linguistic affinity can be seen among many of the names, for instance, consider *malohu, maloku, amaloku, malop, malok, malk, malox, malou, namaluk, namaloku*, and *nmalok*. Other names on the list include *nigui, nga, naga, gwie, miau, mia*, and *mio*. Although the distribution of kava in New Guinea is very erratic, as discussed later, authors and ethnobotanists have recorded a very large number of vernacular names for the plant (Lebot and Cabalion, 1988). Some of those encountered in the literature include *koi* and *keu* from the north-east, *gamoda, gamada*, and *komata* from the Fly River estuary, *wati* from the Marind-Anim in the western province, *toe, towe, toa*, and *tigwa* from southern New Guinea, and *bari, tigwa, ikawati*, and *wati* from West Papua and western Papua New Guinea.

Ethnobotanical studies show that there are considerable differences in the selection and use of particular cultivars (Lebot and Cabalion, 1988). Some are used only for ceremonial purposes, others in the treatment of medical disorders with particular cultivars being used for specific ailments and complaints, and the largest number, of course, for regular drinking (Lebot and Brunton, 1985). Thus, the differences observed are of great ethno-botanical interest in terms of their significance in the communities which recognize and use them.

The physiological effects of kava produced upon consumption is a major factor in its traditional selection and use. Cultivars which produce less than desirable effects may not be replanted, while the stem cuttings from those that are favored because they are outstanding in some way are used for clone propagation and distribution. According to

Lebot and Lévesque (1989), "...very few other species have been subjected to such selection pressure on individual plants. This attention comes to bear first on the chemical composition, which is directly responsible for the physiological effect felt by the drinker, rather than on morphological characters."

Lebot and Lévesque (1989) state that the current vernacular names assigned to the cultivars are associated with the plant's morphological descriptions, and sometimes the region where the cultivar is thought to have originated. Davis and Brown (1999), however, contend that besides the morphological characteristics of the plant, which in their description are even more detailed than those provided by Lebot and Lévesque (1996), and the geographical origin, kava growers also distinguish cultivars on the basis of certain ancillary characteristics, such as the smell and taste of the beverage, and its physiological (psychoactive) effects on drinkers. The morphological features listed by Davis and Brown (1999) in their classification scheme include:

1. plant stature (e.g., erect, prostrate, dwarf, regular),
2. relative internode length and thickness (e.g., short and thin, short and thick, long and thin, long and thick),
3. lenticel distribution on stems (e.g., regularly or irregularly spaced),
4. stem color (e.g., light or dark green, dark green with a purple tinge),
5. leaf color (e.g., light or dark green, yellow, green with a purple tinge),
6. leaf pubescence or hairiness.

For instance, in Fiji the cultivar name *vula kasa leka* means "white with short internodes" (where *vula* = white; *kasa* = internode; *leka* = short). Thus, traditional Fijian cultivars have a name related to their phenotype (e.g., in addition to those listed above, *damu* = red; *loa* = black; *balavu* = long; *matakaro* = spotted; *Qila* is a well-known village on the Fijian island of Taveuni where this cultivar most likely originated). Under the traditional system of classification, about 15 cultivars were known in Fiji at the beginning of the twentieth century (Parham, 1935; Steinmetz, 1960). A key developed by farmers there and based on morphological features allowed for efficient differentiation among the cultivars. Lebot and Lévesque (1989) listed 27 sample cultivars they collected and subsequently assayed for their kavalactone or kavapyrone content (see Table 6 therein). Besides *vula kasa leka*, other cultivars listed include *vula kasa balavu*, *matakaro balavu*, *qila leka*, *qila balavu*, *business*, and *honolulu*. The last two may be newly introduced cultivars, and indicate the dynamic nature of cultivar dispersal. Steinmetz's (1960) description of "white variety, kasa leka," probably *vula kasa leka*, is typical and exemplary of the five most cultivated "varieties" of that time: "White variety, *kasa leka* – the stems are about 3–5 cm in diameter, the branches leave fairly wide scars of about 2.5 cm, the internodes are short (5–7 cm) and the stem is green, with lentil-sized spotting."

After a later survey, Lebot *et al.* (1997) have concluded that kava in Fiji (except for Lau Group and Rotuma) is represented by eleven cultivars (eleven morphotypes). They give the following descriptions for *vula kasa leka* and some other varieties:

Vula kasa leka – Light green; short internodes with many dark green spots; prostrate general appearance; pubescence on the edge of the lamina which is opened, regular, and pale green.

Loa kasa balavu – Dark purple stem; long thin internodes with many lenticels; generally normal appearance with no leaf pubescence; regular dark-green laminae with a purple tinge on the insert point of the petiole.

Loa kasa leka – Dark purple stem; short thick internodes with many lenticels; generally normal appearance with no leaf pubescence; regular dark-green laminae with a purple tinge on the insert point of the petiole.

Qila balavu – Dark green stems with long, thick internodes and many spots; erect general appearance; pubescence on the edge of the drooping, elongated, dark-green laminae.

Honolulu – Long, thin internodes that are light green with few dark green spots on the upper parts but uniform with a dark green tinge on the lower parts; regular, round, pale-green laminae with no pubescence; normal general appearance.

It should be noted that for the commercial exploitation of kava in Fiji, only two cultivars, *loa kasa leka* and *loa kasa balavu*, are commonly planted. The selection is made because they are known for their general hardiness, disease resistance, faster maturity, and a higher crop yield, not necessarily because they produce the best or most palatable beverage.

Fijian farmers and drinkers of the beverage also distinguish among the organs of the plant. The *waka* (the lateral roots and rootlets) is the most favored and fetches the highest commercial price, then *lewena* (the thickened underground parts of the stem or stump, sometimes incorrectly called the rhizome), and lastly *kasa* (the first few nodes and internodes of the stem). In the late 1990s, the average market price (US currency per kg) in Fiji was \$12 for *waka*, \$8 for *lewena*, and \$4–5 for *kasa*. This gradation may have arisen from and may be directly related to the kavalactone content of the different plant parts which, according to Smith (1983), is highest in the *waka* and least in the *kasa*.

In Tonga, the traditional classification system, which is similar to that in Fiji, is based on a choice between two characters, first the color, then the shape of the internode. Cultivar names, some of which are binomial, reflect morphological characteristics, for example, *akau* for long internodes, *fulufulu* for hairy, *hina* for white or light green, *huli* for black or purple, *leka* for short internodes, and *valu* for eight. Altogether, eight cultivars have been identified by Lebot *et al.* (1997), namely: *ata, hina, hina 'akau, kula, kula 'akau, lau fulufulu* (or *lau fulufalua*), *leka kula*, and *valu*. Davis and Brown (1999) have identified a ninth cultivar called *leka hina*. In Samoa, five cultivars are normally recognized. Three of them, *ava talo, ava mumu*, and *ava sa*, are relatively uncommon. The other two, *ava lea* and *ava la'au*, are the most popular and frequently cultivated. Only three cultivars are recognized on the Polynesians islands of Wallis and Futuna, namely, *huli kata loa, hina kata loa*, and *hina leka*. As in other countries, cultivar names relate to distinctive morphological features, for instance, *hina* for white, *huli* for black, *loa* for long, and *kata* for internode.

Cultivar classification systems in Vanuatu vary from community to community and result from detailed observations of variations between and within clones. The village elders usually are the repository of such information, and appear to have had this function for a long time. Vanuatu has over 100 recorded vernacular languages and dialects, and kava and its cultivars possess a name in most of them. Cultivar names, in accordance with Vanuatu's traditional classification system (Cabalion and Morat, 1983), often consist of a "big name," equivalent of the generic name, followed by a "small name" or the name of the particular cultivar, thus forming a double, analogous to the binomial of the Linnaean system. On some islands, however, there often is just one name for each cultivar.

Lebot *et al.* (1997) describe 19 cultivars from Pentecost and 16 from Tanna, with the two islands together comprising the two main diversification areas for kava in Vanuatu.

Some of the cultivar names in Apma language from Melsisi area of central Pentecost are as follows:

Borogu – The stems of this cultivar have a regular thickness and are brown, but turn green at the ends. The leaves have a fairly pale green hue, but turn dark when cultivated in a coastal or forest site. In dry areas, the ends of the leaves display a yellow tinge. They measure about 15 cm long and 10 cm wide. The internodes vary in length between 15 and 20 cm. Kava drink produced from this cultivar is slightly bitter but quite strong, and a single cupful produces the desired effect.

Boro means "small in size." The root mass of the cultivar is fairly compact and does not grow deep, but rather spreads out at a shallow depth. This cultivar is the drinker's favorite in Pentecost.

Borogu is called *borogoru* in the north of the island and *gorogoro* in the south.

Melmel – This cultivar produces very fine stems and branches and small yellow leaves. Kava drink made from it has very feeble effects; thus it is called *melmel*, which means "nothing." No after effects are felt the day following consumption, even if large quantities are consumed. Usually it is reserved for chiefs because it allows them to carry on drinking kava while talking for extended periods of time without losing control of their muscles and nodding off to sleep. The *melmel* cultivar is a small plant, under 2 m tall, with internodes 20 to 25 cm long.

Bogong – This form of *P. wichmannii* is not cultivated but grows wild in the forest. *Bogong* means "big and strong." In the north it is called *bogongo*; in the south, *liap*.

Malmalbo – *Malmal* means "rotten." The taste and smell of this cultivar are reminiscent of rotten pig meat. It produces a highly potent beverage, and drinkers experience its effects over two or three days. The cultivar is fairly uncommon and is used mainly in traditional medicine to relieve rheumatic pains. Its stems are paler than those of *borogu* and its leaves smell like those of *melmel* or *bukulit*. The laminae are a darker green than those of *borogu*.

Names of some cultivars used in central Tanna are as follows:

Pia – The name of this cultivar means "smooth" or "hairless," referring to the appearance of the internodes. The beverage produced from it is the kava of reconciliation, traditionally used to settle disputes and misunderstandings or to appease angry ancestors and spirits.

Ahouia – The stump of this cultivar has a very distinct yellow interior (*ahouia* means "yellow"), indicating that it is very potent and rich in kavalactone content.

Apin – Meaning "black," the name of this cultivar refers to its dark purplish-blue stems. It grows very slowly, is not very popular and mainly used to treat rheumatism. *Apin* is believed to be a magical kava. Thus, it is also planted close to the sacred area of the *nakamal* (kava-drinking area) where drinkers spit *tamafa* or kava libations to their ancestors.

Rhowen – The name refers to the white stems of the plant, which in fact are very pale green in color. The beverage prepared from this cultivar is drunk to guard against sorcery.

Unlike in Fiji, Vanuatu farmers do not differentiate among the organs of the plant for commercial value or quality of the beverage prepared from them. A rigorous description and complete inventory of the vernacular names applied in Vanuatu to

P. methysticum cultivars, together with their cultural significance, is contained in an excellent monograph by Lebot and Cabalion (1988).

In Tahiti, 14 cultivars were recorded by Cuzent (1860) who provided vernacular names, uses, and morphological descriptions for each. He mentioned that the strength or weakness of the beverage obtained from the cultivars were the main characteristics used by the native Tahitians to classify them. He also stated that the chemical characteristics were more important than the morphological features to the users. Brown (1935) noted that in the Marquesas islands "the species were intentionally cultivated by the natives, who had selected 21 varieties differing in the height, length, and color of the internodes, the size of the leaves, and in chemical composition." Although efforts by Christian missionaries and colonizers to eradicate kava from these societies were largely successful, relict plants of past cultivation were located by Lebot during surveys in 1987 in the thick wet forest in French Polynesia.

As Titcomb (1948) has indicated, kava use in Hawai'i survived into early twentieth century, and after that continued to grow as relict populations in a number of steep-sided, shady valleys on some of the islands. Handy (1940) described 14 cultivars from Hawai'i which had previously been recognized. While his brief descriptions do not permit us to reconstruct a reliable traditional classification system, they are nonetheless informative. For example:

Ap – Has long joints and dark green stalk.

Liwa – Is distinguished by short joints and green stalk.

Makea – Has long internodes and is lighter green than *apu*.

Mo'i – The internodes are short and dark green, and the nodes are somewhat whitish.

Papa – Has short internodes and spotted stalk.

The situation in Hawai'i is similar to most other places where kava use has declined or disappeared in that many vernacular names have been lost as other names no longer in use can be located in historical documents and other reference materials (Lebot and Lévesque, 1989).

Plant Morphology

Piper methysticum is a member of the pepper or Piperaceae family, order Piperales, class Dicotyledonae. The pepper family includes more than 2,000 species of herbs, shrubs, small trees, and woody climbers distributed throughout the tropics (Heywood, 1978). The leaves of Piperaceae usually are alternate, entire, and petiolate, with the flowers uniformly small and grouped on a dense spike.

Of the several hundred species that comprise the genus *Piper*, about ten yield food or medicinal drugs useful to humans. They include pepper (*P. nigrum* L.), the commonly used spice; betel (*P. betle* L.), indigenous to India and Southeast Asia and whose leaves are used with areca nut as masticatories; the long peppers (*P. officinarum* C. DC. and *P. longum* L.), distributed throughout the Indian subcontinent and used as spices; and, of course, *P. methysticum*.

Piper methysticum is a robust, fairly succulent, well-branching, perennial shrub or bush which adopts an erect posture with an upright, ramifying stem (Figure 1.1 and Figure 4.1) resembling other Piperaceae. When cultivated, the plant is usually harvested when it is 2–3 m tall, but in warm and humid conditions and with enough

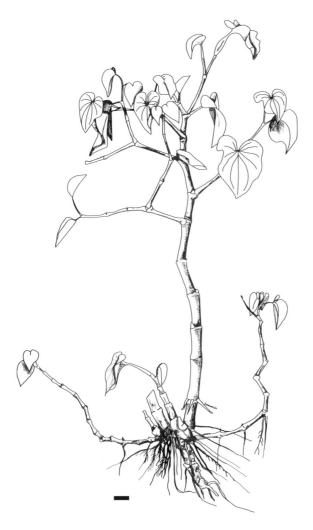

Figure 4.1 Piper methysticum Forst. f. drawing showing the general appearance of the kava plant. Calibration bar equals 4 cm. Reproduced from Lebot and Lévesque (1989) *Allertonia*, 5(2), 223–280, with permission from the National Tropical Botanical Garden.

sunlight, it grows densely to heights above 6 m (Singh, 1992). By this time, it would have reached senescence at an age of 15–20 years, depending on cultivar type.

Branches and stems are glabrous and fleshy. The stems are usually between 2 and 4 cm in diameter at the internode and develop from a crown which is 10–40 cm wide at the neck. Side branches develop from the young parts of the stem and, with age, they die and fall away leaving distinctive scars on the nodes.

Depending on the cultivar or variety, branches sprout from the stem in a dextrogyrate or levogyrate arrangement. On reaching maturity, the plant's general appearance is that of a bouquet of woody stems clustered together at the base. The plant does not produce many leaves. Those that it does are thin, single, heart-shaped, alternate, and quite large, being 8–25 cm long and sometimes wider than they are long (Figure 4.2). They

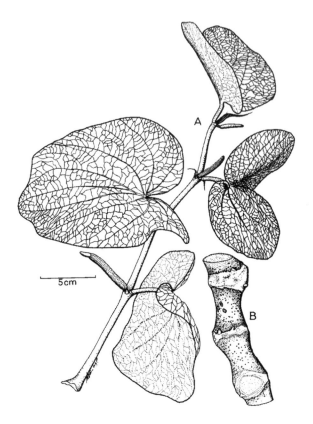

Figure 4.2 A. Habit of a kava branch collected near Suva, Fiji. B. Part of stem of a mature plant
showing the internodes and the swollen nodes. Reprinted from Singh (1992) Kava, an
overview, *Journal of Ethnopharmacology*, 37, 13–45, with permission from Elsevier Science.

are deciduous and rot quickly, being carried on petioles that are 2–6 cm in length.
Although generally smooth, some varieties show a very fine pubescence on the underside
and occasionally the upper surface of the lamina or the veins. The inflorescence, axillary
to or opposite the leaves, is a spadix typical of the Piperaceae. The flowers are small and
unisexual, and are closely bunched around a rigid axis (Figure 4.3). The species is dioecious,
so that the male flowers with their stamens are found on one plant and the female flowers
with pistils on another.

As previously mentioned, *P. methysticum* is incapable of sexual reproduction and
depends almost entirely on human intervention for its vegetative propagation. Once a
stem cutting is planted, new growth occurs at a stem bud at the axil of a lateral branch
scar. An upright shoot grows and then axillary buds and lateral axes appear. A root system
develops from the underground part of the stem cutting and this feeds the stem cutting
leading to the growth and development of the stump and the aerial parts of the plant.

Kava is cultivated primarily for its rootstock, also referred to as the stump, where the
highest levels of the kavalactones are located. Kava is also harvested for its stalks.
The stump has often been incorrectly referred to as a rhizome. A true rhizome is a horizontally creeping underground stem that bears leafy roots – an organ usually found in

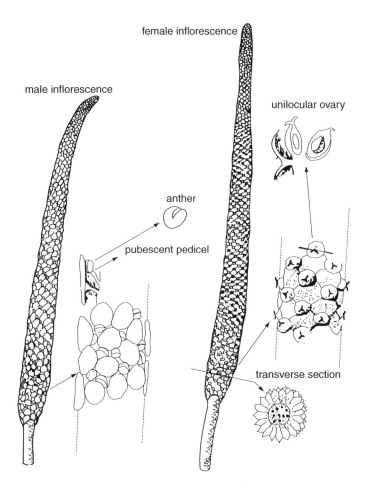

female inflorescence

male inflorescence

unilocular ovary

anther

pubescent pedicel

transverse section

Figure 4.3 Piper methysticum Forst. f. male and female inflorescences. Reproduced from Lebot and Lévesque (1989) *Allertonia*, 5(2), 223–280, with permission from the National Tropical Botanical Garden.

monocotyledons (Lebot *et al.*, 1997). *P. methysticum* has no rhizomes, but bears monopodial stems with sympodial branches which grow from the stem. The stump is knotty, thick, sometimes tuberous, and often contains holes or cracks due to partial destruction of the parenchyma, especially as it ages. A fringe of lateral roots up to 2–3 m long extends from the spongy and pithy rootstock (Figure 2.3). The roots comprise a large number of ligneous fibers and consist of 60–70% starch. The rootstock varies in color from white to dark yellow depending on the kavalactone content in the plant resin. Under cultivation, the kava rootstock develops as a large radiating, starchy mass as a result of intensive soil mounding and other planting techniques developed by generations of farmers growing Pacific root crops.

Based on agronomic surveys conducted in Vanuatu and Fiji, the average fresh weight of kava root system is found to be about 1 kg at the age of 10–12 months. The average number of stems or stalks is 11, and the number of nodes on the longest stem is about 10 (Lebot and Cabalion, 1988; Y.N. Singh, unpublished observations). Depending on cultivar and stage of maturity, the fresh weight can be up to 50 kg, although exceptionally large specimens have been encountered. For instance, a four-year-old plant grown in very sandy soil in Port Vila, Vanuatu, had a fresh stump weight of 132 kg when uprooted by Lebot (Lebot and Cabalion, 1988). On air drying in the sun by the traditional method, the final product usually is about 2–10% of the original fresh weight.

Taxonomy and Nomenclature

The date when *P. methysticum* was first recognized by European explorers is unknown, however, the Dutch navigators Le Maire and Schouten reported its presence on Wallis and Futuna Islands as early as 1616 (Brosses, 1756). Thus, kava was probably familiar to travellers to the Pacific at the time of the first voyage of Captain James Cook on the HMS *Endeavour* (1768–71). Cook showed particular interest in the plant, including methods of the beverage preparation, the related ceremonies, and its importance in the social structure of the indigenous communities. While accompanying Cook on his first voyage, Sydney Parkinson, the artist charged with the task of making drawings of newly discovered plants, recorded and made one of the first drawings of the plant. This drawing is preserved in the Natural History section of the British Museum, London, England (Figure 1.4). They named the plant *P. inebrians*, from the Latin *inebriare* (to intoxicate). However, the credit for the first detailed description of the plant for taxonomic purposes is normally given to Johann G.A. Forster (Forster, 1777) who joined Cook's second voyage (1772–75) as a botanist, along with his father J.R. Forster. Forster named the kava plant with the binomial *P. methysticum* or "intoxicating pepper," *péperi* being Greek for "peppery" or "pungent," *methysticum* being the Latin transcription of the Greek *methustikos* and derived from *methu* which, according to Steinmetz (1960), means "intoxicating drink."

Botanical synonyms of *P. methysticum* include *Macropiper methysticum* Miquel, *P. decumanum* Optiz, *P. inebrians* Scholander ex Parkinson and Bertero, and *P. spurium* Forst. Related species have been identified in a number of places, for instance, *P. torricellense* Lauterb. from New Guinea (Burkill, 1935; Sterly, 1970), *P. puberulum* Benth., the so-called "Honolulu kava," *P. excelsum* Forster, from New Zealand, known to the native Maoris as kawa or kawa-kawa but without the properties of *P. methysticum* and whose leaves were used by them in the past in an infusion for headaches (Steinmetz, 1960), *P. plantageum* Schlechter, native to Mexico and used there in the same manner as *P. excelsum*, and *P. latifolium*, synonymous with *M. latifolium* Forster (Forster, 1777), endemic to Oceania and used in the native pharmacopoeia of Vanuatu (Vienne, 1981).

Collected specimens in herbaria, museums, and those examined by various botanists had no seeds, and female flowers were uncommon. Degener (1940) had not seen a single female plant in any of the many plantations he had visited in Hawai'i and noted that other colleagues had been unable to describe any in their accounts because none could be found. However, a few publications give descriptions of seeds but no herbarium specimens are cited, making verification of this information impossible (Lebot and Lévesque, 1989). Experience of native farmers in the Pacific confirms the opinion that *P. methysticum* does not bear fruit. In Vanuatu, farmers are unanimous in that they have never seen fruits or seeds on any kava plants. However, Lebot and Lévesque (1989) claim that *P. methysticum* does flower. It is dioecious, and produces both male and female inflorescences on separate plants, but does not reproduce sexually. When hand pollinated, female inflorescences fall off before they can bear fruit. Weather and insects are the natural vectors for pollination in the Piperaceae family (Semple, 1974). If pollination is successful, the small fruits are dispersed by the wind, by falling to the ground, or by birds and bats. In the case of *P. methysticum*, wind-pollination is unlikely because the sticky, glutinous pollen is not easily washed off or blown away.

Botanic Origins

The botanic origins of kava have been of considerable interest both to anthropologists and ethnobotanists. This is because *P. methysticum* is always propagated vegetatively, and thus the identification of its wild ancestor may indicate its area of origin and help to trace the ancient migration patterns of kava-using peoples of the Pacific. According to Lebot *et al.* (1997), there is little evidence to suggest that kava is indigenous to Polynesia as none of the *Piper* species in this area is closely related morphologically to *P. methysticum*. From a botanical viewpoint, it is considered that the greatest incidence of allied species in a specific area is a good indicator of the origin of a plant. Since the number of *Piper* species is most heavily concentrated in Melanesia, Lebot *et al.* (1997) have proposed that kava was domesticated somewhere in this region.

Other botanists have also considered the origin of *P. methysticum*. Yuncker (1959) concluded that, "...its origin is problematical...," and according to Smith (1981), "the nativity of *Piper methysticum* is uncertain, but probably...was indigenous in eastern Melanesia or possibly in the New Hebrides (*now called Vanuatu*); it is now widely cultivated eastward throughout the Pacific and is occasionally naturalized. It is certainly one of the first plants that aboriginal voyagers would have taken with them." An earlier suggestion that *M. latifolium* might be the Melanesian precursor of kava has been discounted, given the significant chemical and morphological differences between the two genera (Smith, 1975). Cuzent's (1857) claim that Tahitians used *M. latifolium* to prepare the kava drink almost certainly referred to *P. methysticum*. Furthermore, *M. latifolium* roots contain no psychoactive kavalactones, and its major chemical constituent is β-asarone, a central nervous system depressant (Lebot *et al.*, 1997).

A number of other possible ancestors of kava exist within the *Piper* genus. Two which are closely related to *P. methysticum* are endemic to northern Melanesia, namely, *P. wichmannii* C. DC. (whose synonyms include *P. erectum* C. DC., *P. schlechteri* C. DC., and *P. arbuscula* Trealease) and *P. gibbilimbum* C. DC. *P. wichmannii* C. DC. (Figure 4.4) is commonly found in Papua New Guinea, the Solomon Islands, and northern Vanuatu, particularly at elevations around 800 m, while *P. gibbilimbum* has successfully colonized disturbed forests in Papua New Guinea. Lebot *et al.* (1997) have also raised the outside possibility that *P. methysticum* arose as a hybrid of related *P.* species. For example, *P. methysticum* could be a sterile (F_1) interspecific hybrid of *P. wichmannii* and *P. gib-bilimbum*, both of which reproduce sexually. However, field observations by these authors suggest that hybrids of the two species do not occur. Their plants are often found growing close to each other without any obvious signs of hybridization.

A number of other lines of evidence point to the reproductively fertile *P. wichmannii* C. DC. as the most likely wild progenitor of *P. methysticum*. The natural habitat of *P. wickmannii* is dense rain forest with persistent foliage. Like *P. methysticum*, it is a shade-loving species whose distribution as a wild or cultivated plant is restricted to wet equatorial or subtropical climates between 25° north latitude and 25° south latitude (Lebot *et al.*, 1997). Thus, the area of origin of *P. methysticum* lies somewhere within the range of distribution of *P. wickmannii*, an area including New Guinea, the Solomon Islands, and the northern part of Vanuatu (Chew, 1972). The large number of varieties of *P. methysticum* found in northern Vanuatu, the occurrence there of *P. wickmannii*, and other lines of evidence suggest that location as the center (or the most important center) of domestication of *P. methysticum* (Lebot *et al.*, 1997). According to Chew (1972), *P. wichmannii* is the most closely related taxon to *P. methysticum*. Morphological differences between them in coloration and pigmentation of stem internodes, leaf coloring or pubescence on lamina, woody elements of roots, etc., are no more significant than those among different cultivars of *P. methysticum*. The major morphological difference between the two taxa is the length of the inflorescence. The inflorescence of *P. wichmannii* is as long as the lamina – 15 to 30 cm. That of *P. methysticum* varies between 6 and 20 cm, but is always shorter than the lamina (Figures 4.2 and 4.4). In fact, native farmers in Vanuatu who are able to distinguish many cultivars on the basis of morphological features consider that forms of *P. methysticum* and *P. wichmannii* belong to the same species and identify both these plants as kava, and even experienced botanists occasionally

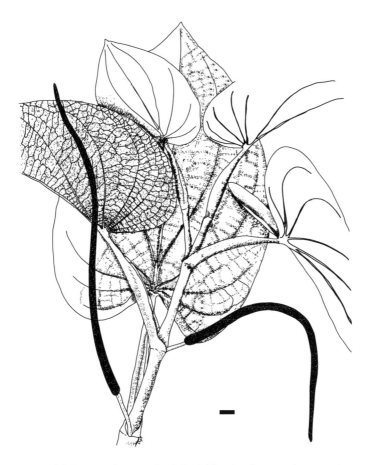

Figure 4.4 Piper wichmannii C. DC. Calibration bar equals 2 cm. Reproduced from Lebot and Lévesque (1989) *Allertonia*, 5(2), 223–280, with permission from the National Tropical Botanical Garden.

confuse the two. Only one other significant difference exists between the two taxa, that in root characteristics. The tissue of *P. wichmannii* is noticeably harder and the proportion of woody elements is higher than that in *P. methysticum*.

A survey of genetic resources of kava in the Pacific has revealed the extent of genetic diversity existing within kava and between *P. methysticum* and *P. wichmannii* (Lebot and Lévesque, 1989). There was appreciable variability among cultivars, both in morphology and kavalactone composition and content. The morphological variability in growth habit, internode color, and lamina shape and pigmentation has permitted 118 different kava clones to be distinguished. This diversity was attributed to the effect of natural selection operating under different climatic and ecological conditions in the island countries. However, no clear relationship was observed between the phenotypic variation and the geographic locations, a situation that probably arose largely as a result of human dispersal of the plant.

A relatively recent introduction to some of the main kava-growing areas of the South Pacific is what has been named "false kava." This term is applied to plants that resemble the genuine kava but which lack the kavalactones and the associated kava odor. It has not been established whether these plants are cultivars of *P. methysticum* or constitute a different species of *Piper* (Davis and Brown, 1999).

False kava has been reported from Fiji, French Polynesia, Hawai'i, Pohnpei, Samoa, Tonga, and Vanuatu. The main false kava species is *P. auritum*, which occurs in Hawai'i and (since late 1998 or early 1999) in Pohnpei. Outside of the South Pacific, *P. auritum* extends from southern Mexico to northern South America and South Florida. In Fiji, false kava is mostly *P. aduncum* and is known locally as *yaqona ni onolulu*. Whether it is in any way related to the *honolulu* cultivar of *P. methysticum* described earlier is not yet clear. *Yaqona ni onolulu* was first recorded in Fiji in 1924 and is suspected to have arrived in packing materials at Suva port by ship, and appears to have spread out from Suva along roadsides. In Vanuatu, false kava is attributed to *P. wickmannii* and *P. aduncum*. In Tonga, the plant is said to have originated in Hawai'i and is called *kava Hawai'i*. On the Samoan island of Upolu, it is believed to have come from Fiji in about 1994 and is named *'ava Fiti*.

The large 20–50 cm leaves of *P. auritum* are borne into alternate ranks and are often held horizontally on horizontal upper branches, thus forming a broad light-intercepting crown with relatively few, large, pale green leaves. The flowering spikes are typically 18–20 cm long. Leaves and roots have a characteristic odor similar to aniseed or sarsaparilla. It is less branched than *P. methysticum* giving a characteristic appearance to a colony with many vertical stems and few branches. This differs from kava, which typically grows in individual clumps. False kava sprouts prolifically from rhizomes and also roots from nodes, leading to rapid spreading. The stems of *P. auritum* do not exhibit the characteristic swollen nodes of genuine kava (Figure 4.2). *P. auritum* grows very rapidly, to heights greater than genuine kava and exceeding six meters. *P. aduncum* is a tree up to six meters tall with leaves up to 15 cm long and flowers borne on cream-colored drooping spikes about 12–13 cm long.

There are two major problems posed by false kava. First, it can be harvested and mixed intentionally or unintentionally with genuine kava and in this way reduces the quality of the product. This practice could have a serious impact on the regional and overseas export markets. Second, because it is larger than genuine kava and grows more vigorously, it can be a weed that interferes with the growth of other crops. It may also be an alternate host and harbor pests and pathogens of kava, although this has yet to be demonstrated.

Interaction of Environment, Ontogeny and Chemotypes of Kava

Chemotype variation within cultivars (see Chapter 5) from Vanuatu was evaluated by Lebot and Lévesque (1989, 1996). Specimens of the same cultivar growing in different soils and under varying climatic environments were harvested and analyzed, whilst different cultivars of differing origins were grown in the same environment and harvested together. Results showed that there was considerable variation in total kava-lactone content between cultivars, indicating that chemical composition and total kavalactone content is controlled by the genotype rather than by external environmental factors. This confirmed the previous ethnobotanical results of Lebot and Cabalion (1986) who reported the assertions by farmers that different cultivars uprooted from the same garden on the same day produced different physiological effects. In other words, when different cultivars from both *P. wichmannii* and *P. methysticum* are planted in a similar environment, they produce a range of chemotypes. However, when a culti-var is cloned, the resultant plant displays a homogenous chemotype and kavalactone content very similar to the parent plant. A trial was carried out with *Vila* and *Small leaf* in which clones of these two cultivars were planted on the same day and harvested exactly two years later. The clones displayed similar kavalactone content and the chemotypes remained homogenous among clones, including the parent plant of each cultivar (Lebot and Lévesque, 1989, 1996). In addition, samples of the same cultivars collected from different Fijian islands displayed very similar chemotypes despite their different envir-onmental origins (Lebot and Lévesque, 1989).

Lebot and Lévesque (1989) also conducted several trials on two different Pacific islands to examine the effect of ontogeny on kava chemotype. Kavalactone content was highest after an average of 18 months and the content remained stable during the subsequent growth of the plant, although the rootstock biomass continued to increase over time. Clones from different cultivars were planted in a row on the same day and one plant from each cultivar was harvested every five months. Plants grown for the trials on Santo Island (altitude 140 m; average annual precipitation 3,200 mm) were compared with control plants selected from the local village garden and also with the same cultivar from the germplasm collection on Éfate Island (altitude 40 m; average annual precipitation 2,400 mm). Results showed that the kavalactone content was not related to ontogeny but rather to the genotype. However, some cultivars such as *Marino* and *Malogro* displayed very consistent chemotypes, whereas other cultivars like *Tudey* appeared to be subject to great variation (Lebot and Lévesque, 1989, 1996).

Chemotypes do not always correspond to the morphological characteristics of cultivars that are considerably variable. In some cases plants with similar morphotypes also have similar chemotypes, but exceptions are numerous (Lebot and Lévesque, 1989). Absence of a consistent correlation between chemotype and morphotype is probably reflective of the farmers' attention being focused on the chemical content rather than on the morphological characteristics of the kava cultivars. This may also account in part for the retention of the morphological similarity of *P. methysticum* to its probable wild progenitor *P. wichmannii* (Lebot and Lévesque, 1989). On the basis of data obtained from these trials and the statements made by farmers, it may be inferred that Vanuatu possesses the *in situ* collections of the different clones produced from the domestication process of *P. wichmannii*. Among these clones, some are replicants and others are variants of given chemotypes. By selecting appropriate variants, farmers have developed the cultivated species *P. methysticum*, which is rich in kavain and poor in dihydrokavain, from its wild progenitor *P. wichmannii*, which is rich in dihydrokavain and poor in kavain (Lebot and Lévesque, 1989). A schematic lineage of chemotypes was proposed by Lebot and Lévesque (1989), as illustrated in Figure 4.5, demonstrating the development of the cultivated *P. methysticum* from *P. wichmannii*. As mentioned earlier, the evidence suggests that the center of origin and diversification of *P. methysticum* was probably the northern part of Vanuatu. From there, Polynesian travellers may have spread clones to other Pacific islands. This hypothesis may also explain why *P. methysticum* is not present in the Solomon Islands (Lebot and Lévesque, 1989).

Distribution of Chemotypes

Chemotypes of cultivars from throughout the Pacific islands were grouped in alphabetical order (A–I) by a multivariant analysis of chemical contents of the cultivars (Lebot and Lévesque, 1989) (Figure 4.6). Chemotypes in groups A, B, C, and D, all exclusive to Melanesia, are variants of *P. wichmannii* typified by very low kavain content. Of these, *vambu*, *buara*, *bo*, *kau*, and *kau kupwe* are cultivated from Vanuatu and Baluan (Papua New Guinea). Chemotypes in group A and B have high proportions of dihydromethysticin (38–58%) and dihydrokavain. These two kavalactones together account for approximately 64–75% of the total kavalactone content. The proportion of kavain content in these two groups is relatively low (<3%) (Lebot and Lévesque, 1989). Chemotype C is represented by only one wild form of *P. wichmannii* from the Madang area of Papua New Guinea, and has high concentrations of dihydrokavain, and dihydromethysticin and very low proportion of kavain. Chemotype D has approximately equal proportions of dihydrokavain, dihydromethysticin, and methysticin (31, 30, and 27%, respectively) and little kavain (1%) (Lebot and Lévesque, 1989). Chemotypes in groups E, F, G, H, and I occur predominantly in cultivars of *P. methysticum*. These chemotypes are found in Melanesia, Polynesia, and Micronesia. Group E chemotypes from Vanuatu, Wallis and Futuna, Hawai'i, Tonga, Marquesas, and the Carolines produce beverages with strong physiological effects resulting from very high proportions of dihydrokavain and dihydromethysticin (Lebot and Lévesque, 1989). Chemotypes in group F are distributed exclusively in Papua New Guinea and Vanuatu. All kava cultivars in Papua New Guinea exhibit this unique group of chemotypes. Group F chemotypes, similar to those of chemotypes in group E, are rich in dihydrokavain and dihydro-methysticin but have low levels of yangonin. Chemotypes of this group do not produce a desirable psychoactive effect. Cultivars of this group are, therefore, not used for daily consumption. Chemotypes in groups G, H, and I are widely distributed through out Polynesia, Fiji, and Vanuatu and are rich in kavain and the most popular kavalactone blends. Chemotype G is known to produce a beverage suitable for daily consumption, especially in Vanuatu and Wallis where the roots are consumed fresh (Lebot and Lévesque, 1989). Chemotype H produces the most palatable beverage and is present only in Vanuatu and Western Samoa (Lebot and Lévesque, 1989). Chemotype I spread throughout Fiji and is present in Tonga, Samoa, Tahiti, Hawai'i, and Pohnpei. Chemotypes in this group are rich in methysticin and kavain (Lebot and Lévesque, 1989).

The chemotypic diversity of kava within Vanuatu is greater than elsewhere in the Pacific, and variability among the cultivars from Pentecost in Vanuatu is as great as

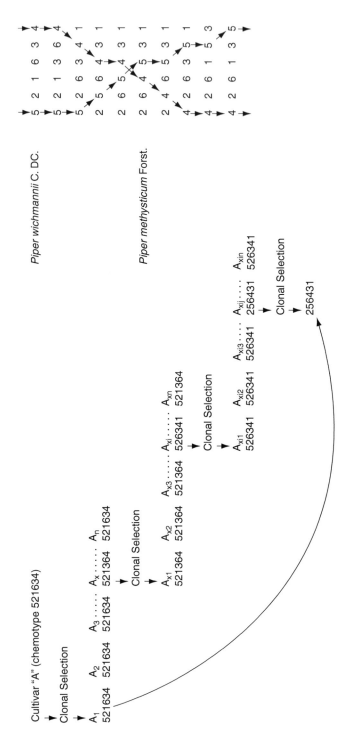

Figure 4.5 Schematic proposal for the development of the cultivated *Piper methysticum*. Domestication of kava was carried out from a chemotype rich in dihydroka-vain and poor in kavain (*P. wichmannii*) to chemotypes rich in kavain and poor in dihydrokavain (*P. methysticum*). Reproduced from Lebot and Lévesque (1989) *Allertonia*, 5(2), 223–280, with permission from the National Tropical Botanical Garden.

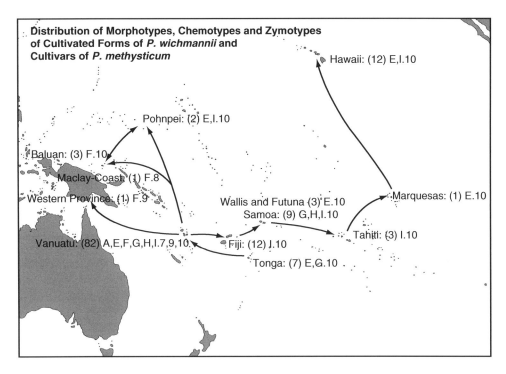

Figure 4.6 Distribution pathways of kava, derived from zymotropic evidence. The numbers in parenthesis
are the number of morphotypes found, the letters indicate chemotype groups, and the numbers
following the letters indicate zymotypes. Reproduced from *Kava, the Pacific Elixir* by Lebot
et al. (1997), with permission from Yale University Press.

that found on all other islands of the Archipelago. All five chemotypes groups (E–I)
selected during the domestication of kava are present today in Vanuatu (Lebot and
Lévesque, 1989).

Genealogy of kava chemotypes studied by Lebot and Lévesque (1989) demonstrates a
domestication process from a truly wild species, which is rich in dihydrokavain, to the
most desirable cultivar which is rich in kavain. These genealogic data support the assertion
that Vanuatu is the country of origin of *P. methysticum*. Moreover, domestication could
not have occurred in Papua New Guinea because of the unsuitable chemotypes of the
wild forms of *P. wichmannii* found in that country. Genealogy also indicates that the
cultivars of *P. methysticum* found in Papua New Guinea today were exported from
Vanuatu early in the domestication process. These cultivars, however, exhibit a modest
improvement in chemical composition, particularly low kavain content. This suggests
an early propagation of kava to a few isolated areas of Papua New Guinea with little
subsequent selection. In contrast, cultivars of Polynesia, probably obtained from northern
Vanuatu, all exhibit improved chemotypes with low percentages of dihydrokavain and
dihydromethysticin. This also holds true for the south of Vanuatu, where the cultivars
of chemotypes A, B, C, and D with high dihydrokavain and dihydromethysticin
contents are absent, confirming a relatively recent introduction of kava from Polynesia,
probably from Samoa (Lebot and Lévesque, 1989). Human dispersal of plant material

has undoubtedly taken place in central Polynesia as well as between Fiji and Tonga, Wallis Island or Samoa. Polynesian travelers passing through Vanuatu selected the most desirable clones. This selection has discouraged the eastward spread of kava of chemotypes A to D and F that possess wilder characteristics (Lebot and Lévesque, 1989).

Interaction between Isozyme and Chemotype of Kava

Genetic research has provided additional evidence suggesting that *P. methysticum* has its ancestral origin in *P. wichmannii* (Lebot *et al.*, 1991). The cultivar assay was used by these workers to determine whether isozymes could be used to characterize and differentiate between cultivars. Polymorphism of isozymes, which are proteins synthesized by genes, serves as a measure of genetic diversity among individuals. Thus, this technique could be applied to assess the degree of genetic diversity within and between *P. methysticum* and *P. wichmannii*, and also to determine whether kava morphotypes from different Pacific islands correspond to different isozyme genotypes (zymotypes). For this study, 25 enzyme systems were assayed, and eight were successfully resolved, including malate dehydrogenase (MDH), aconitase (ACO), phosphoglucomutase (PGM), phosphoglucose isomerase (PGI), isocitrate dehydrogenase (IDH), diaphorase (DIA), malic enzyme (ME), and aldolase (ALD). Analysis of 300 leaf samples revealed that *P. wichmannii* specimens could be grouped into only eight different zymotypes and *P. methysticum* cultivars into just three. Most significantly, one zymotype included individuals from both botanical taxa. The remarkably low isozymic variability among *P. methysticum* cultivars is intriguing – just three zymotypes – when compared to some other common Pacific crops, for example, bananas (*Musa* species), breadfruit (*Artocarpus altilis*), and taro (*Colocasia esculenta*), each of which exhibits over 100 zymotypes in the same geographic area of the Pacific (Lebot *et al.*, 1997). To account for the low level of isozyme variability, they propose that this taxon, *P. methysticum*, consists of sterile clones resulting from human selection of somatic mutants rather than from sexual reproduction, which would have produced a much larger diversity of zymotypes. If this hypothesis is valid then, according to Lebot and co-workers, only a few genes are responsible for the chemical variation among cultivars and none of these are linked with the loci controlling isozyme markers (Lebot *et al.*, 1991; Lebot and Lévesque, 1996). Furthermore, no clear correlation exists between morphotypes and zymotypes since all the Hawaiian cultivars possess the same zymotype, although there are clear morphological and chemical differences (Lebot *et al.*, 1991). Also, the domestication of kava was relatively recent and occurred, as they suggest, in northern Vanuatu. On the other hand, bananas, breadfruit, and taro were domesticated earlier, in Southeast Asia or New Guinea, and spread over a much larger area. Hence human selection for somatic mutants over a longer period of time may account for the greater isozymic variability among these older species. Finally, cytological data from the Lebot *et al.* (1991) study show that both taxa are decaploids with $2n = 10x = 130$ chromosomes, although in *P. methysticum* about a dozen of these chromosomes are four to five times the average size of *P. wichmannii*.

Thus, based on field experience, the length of the inflorescence and the proportion of woody elements in the roots are the only characteristics which allow differentiation between the two taxa. Available botanical data indicate that *P. methysticum* is sterile. Like many cultivated plants, it is a derived form of a fertile wild species. Furthermore, they are the only species in the genus *Piper* from which major psychoactive kavalactones have been isolated (Lebot and Lévesque, 1996). Using field and herbarium observations and cytological and morphological comparisons as data, Lebot *et al.* (1997) concluded that *P. methysticum* is not a separate species but rather is a group of sterile cultivars selected from somatic mutants of *P. wichmannii*. They believe that wild forms of *P. wichmannii* were domesticated and their psychoactive properties improved through active selection of somatic mutants that possessed desirable psychoactive attributes. They propose that *P. methysticum* should be considered not a species but rather a putative cultivar. But kava is such an important economic plant, and subsuming *P. methysticum* within *P. wichmannii* would create both conceptual and practical problems. Thus, as a distinction between wild *P. wichmannii* and cultivated *P. methysticum* is possible and useful, they suggest the following classification:

P. methysticum Forst. f. var. *methysticum*: the sterile, cultivated form.

P. methysticum Forst. f. var. *wichmannii* (DC) Lebot *stat. nov.*: the fertile, wild population.

They also contend that while this classification would not cause any conceptual or practical problems with regard to taxonomy and/or nomenclature, it would, however, allow for ease of communication and differentiation of sterile cultivars and fertile wild populations (Lebot and Lévesque, 1996).

References

Adrian, M. (1996) Substance use and multiculturalism. *Substance Use & Misuse*, 31, 1459–1501.

Barrau, J. (1965) Histoire et préhistoire horticoles de l'Océanie tropicale. *Journal de la Société des Océanistes*, 21, 55–78.

Brosses, C. (1756) *Histoire des Navigations aux Mers Australes*, Chez Durand, Paris. Quoted in Lebot *et al.* (1997).

Brown, F.B.H. (1935) *Flora of Southeastern Polynesia*, Bulletin No. 130, Bernice P. Bishop Museum Press, Honolulu.

Brunton, R. (1989) *The Abandoned Narcotic: Kava and Cultural Instability in Melanesia*, Cambridge University Press, Cambridge.

Burkill, I.H. (1935) *A Dictionary of the Economic Products of the Malay Peninsula*. Scrivener, London.

Cabalion, P. and Morat, P. (1983) Introduction à la végétation, à la flore et aux noms verna-culaires de l'île Pentecôte (Vanuatu). *Journal d'Agriculture Tropicale et de Botanique Appliquée*, 30, 197–248.

Cawte, J. (1985) Psychoactive substances of the South Seas: betel, kava and pituri. *Australian and New Zealand Journal of Psychiatry*, 19, 83–87.

Cawte, J. (1986) Parameters of kava used as a challenge to alcohol. *Australian and New Zealand Journal of Psychiatry*, 20, 70–76.

Chew, W.L. (1972) The genus *Piper* (Piperaceae) in New Guinea, Solomon Islands and Australia. *Journal of the Arnold Arboretum*, 52, 1–25.

Churchill, W. (1916) *Sissano: Movements of Migration within and Through Melanesia*, Carnegie Institution, Washington, DC, pp. 124–144.

Codrington, R.H. (1891) *The Melanesians*. Clarendon, Oxford.

Cuzent, G. (1857) Du kawa ou ava de Tahiti (*Piper methysticum*). *Le Messager de Tahiti* (Papeete), May 10 and November 29.

Cuzent, G. (1860) *Îles de la Société. Tahiti.* Quoted in Lebot and Lévesque (1989).

Davis, R.I. and Brown, J.F. (1999) *Kava* (Piper methysticum) *in the South Pacific: its Importance, Methods of Cultivation, Cultivars, Diseases and Pests*, ACIAR Technical Report No. 46, ACIAR, Canberrra.

Degener, O. (1940) *Flora Hawaiensis*, published privately, Honolulu.

Emerson, O.P. (1903) The Awa Habit of the Hawaiians. *Hawaiian Annual*, pp. 130–140.

Firth, R. (1970) *Rank and Religion in Tikopia*, George Allen and Unwin, London.

Forster, J.G.A. (1777) *A Voyage Around the World in his Britannic Majesty's Sloop* Resolution, Hakluyt Society, London.

Fox, C. (1924) *The Threshold of the Pacific: An Account of the Social Organization, Magic, and Religion of the People of San Cristoval in the Solomon Islands*, K. Paul, Trench and Trubner, London.

Gadjusek, C. (1979) Recent observations on the use of kava, mildly narcotic beverage from New Hebrides. In D. Efron, B. Holmstedt, and N.S. Kline (eds), *Ethnopharmacologic Search for Psychoactive Drugs*, Raven Press, New York, pp. 119–125.

Guiart, J. (1956) Culture contact and the "John Frum" movement in Tanna, New Hebrides. *Southwestern Journal of Anthropology*, 12, 105–116.

Handy, E.S.C. (1927) *Polynesian Religion*, Bulletin No. 34, Bernice P. Bishop Museum Press, Honolulu.

Handy, E.S.C. (1940) *The Hawaiian Planter. Volume 1: His Plants, Methods and Areas of Cultivation*, Bulletin No. 161, Bernice P. Bishop Museum Press, Honolulu, pp. 201–205.

Heywood, V. (ed.) (1978) *Flowering Plants of the World*, Mayflower Books, New York.

Hiroa, T.R. (P. Buck) (1944) *Arts and Crafts of the Cook Islands*, Bulletin No. 179, Bernice P. Bishop Museum Press, Honolulu, pp. 18–20.

Holmes, L.D. (1979) The kava complex in Oceania. *New Pacific*, 4(5), 30–33.

Hood, T.H. (1862) *Notes on a Cruise in H.M.S. Fawn in the Western Pacific*, Edmonston and Douglas, Edinburgh, pp. 20–21, 166.

Krieger, H.W. (1943) *Island Peoples of the Western Pacific*, Smithsonian Institution, Washington DC, p. 22.

Lebot, V. (1991) Kava (*Piper methysticum* Forst. f.): The Polynesian dispersal of an Oceanian plant. In: P. Cox and S. Bannack (eds), *Islands, Plants and Polynesians*, Dioscorides, Portland, OR, pp. 169–201.

Lebot, V. and Brunton, R. (1985) *Tropical Plants as Cash Crops: A Survey of Kava in Vanuatu*, Vanuatu Department of Agriculture, Port Vila.

Lebot, V. and Cabalion, P. (1988) *Kava of Vanuatu: Cultivars of* Piper methysticum *Forst.*, Technical Paper No. 195, South Pacific Commission, Noumea, pp. 1–191.

Lebot, V. and Lévesque, J. (1989) The origin and distribution of kava (*Piper methysticum* Forst. f. and *Piper wichmannii* C. DC., Piperaceae): a phytochemical approach. *Allertonia*, 5, 223–280.

Lebot, V. and Lévesque, J. (1996) Genetic control of kavalactones chemotypes in *Piper methysticum* cultivars. *Phytochemistry*, 43(2), 397–403.

Lebot, V., Aradhya, M. and Manshardt, R.M. (1991) Geographical survey of genetic variation in kava. *Pacific Science*, 45, 169–185.

Lebot, V., Merlin, M. and Lindstrom, L. (1997) *Kava: the Pacific Elixir*, Healing Arts Press, Rochester, VT.

Lester, R.H. (1941) Kava drinking in Vitilevu. *Oceania*, 12, 97–121, 226–254.

Lewin, L. (1924) *Phantastica: Narcotic and Stimulating Drugs*, Routledge, Kegan and Co., London.

Mangeret, R.P. (1884) *Monsigneur Bataillon et les Missions de l'Océanie Centrale*, Vitte et Perrussel, Lyons, pp. 119–126.

Mathews, J.B., Riley, M.D., Fejo, L., Munoz, E., Milns, I., Gardner, J. *et al.* (1988) Effects of the heavy usage of kava on physical health. Summary of a pilot study in an aboriginal community. *Medical Journal of Australia*, 148(11), 548–555.

Métraux, A. (1940) *Ethnology of Easter Island*, Bishop Museum Bulletin, No. 160, Honolulu, p. 159.

Miklouho-Maclay, N. von (1886) Note on the "keu" of the Maclay Coast, New Guinea. *Proceedings of the Linnean Society of New South Wales for 1885*, 10, 687–695.

Moyles, W. (1983) *Aboriginal Community use of Kava as Alcohol Substitute*, Aboriginal Training and Cultural Institute, Balmain, Sydney. Quoted in Cawte (1985).

Newell, N.H. (1947) Kava ceremony in Tonga. *Journey of the Polynesian Society*, 56, 364–417.

Parham, B.E.V. (1935) Wilt disease of yaqona. *Fiji Agriculture Journal*, **8**, 2–8.

Parkinson, S. (1784) *A Journal of a Voyage to the South Seas in his Majesty's Ship, the Endeavour*, S. Parkinson, London, p. 37.

Percy Smith, S. (1920) Kava drinking ceremonies among the Samoans and a boat voyage around 'Upolu, Samoa. *Supplement to the Journal of the Polynesian Society*, **29**(114), 10–13.

Prescott, J. and McCall, G. (eds) (1988) *Kava: Use and Abuse in Australia and the South Pacific*, National Drug and Alcohol Research Centre, University of New South Wales, Sydney, Monograph No. 5.

Rivers, W.H.R. (1914) *The History of the Melanesian Society*, Cambridge University Press, Cambridge.

Schenk, G. (1956) *The Book of Poisons*, Weidenfeld and Nicolson, London.

Semple, K.S. (1974) Pollination in Piperaceae. *Annals of the Missouri Botanical Gardens*, **61**, 868–871.

Singh, Y.N. (1992) Kava: an overview. *Journal of Ethnopharmacology*, **37**, 13–45.

Smiles, S. (1987) Kava, the kava alternative (and why it is stronger in Vanuatu). *Islands Business*, May, pp. 32–33.

Smith, A.C. (1975) The genus *Macropiper* (Piperaceae). *Botanical Journal of the Linnean Society*, **71**, 1–38.

Smith, A.C. (1981) *Flora Vitiensis Nova*, Pacific Tropical Botanical Garden, Kauai.

Smith, R.M. (1983) Kava lactones in *Piper methysticum* from Fiji. *Phytochemistry*, **22**(4), 1055–1056.

Steinmetz, E.F. (1960) Piper methysticum *(Kava)*, Published by the author, Amsterdam.

Sterly, J. (1970) *Heilpflanzen der Einwohner Melanesiens. Beitrage zur Ethnobotanik des Sudwestlichen Pacifik. Hamburger Reihe zur Kultur und Sprachwissenschaft* 6, Hamburg, München.

Thomson, B. (1902) *Savage Island: An Account of a Sojourn in Niue and Tonga*, J. Murray, London, pp. 95–97.

Thomson, B. (1908) *The Fijians. A Study in the Decay of Custom*, Heinemann, London.

Thomson, W.J. (1889) *Te Pito te Henua, or Easter Island*, Smithsonian Institution, Washington, DC, p. 464.

Titcomb, M. (1948) Kava in Hawai'i. *Journal of the Polynesian Society*, **57**, 105–171.

Turner, G. (1861) *Nineteen Years in Polynesia*, J. Snow, London, pp. 122–123

Vienne, B. (1981) *Les usages médicinaux de quelques plantes communes de la flore des îles Banks, Vanuatu*. Quoted in Lebot and Cabalion (1988).

Williamson, R.W. (1939) *Essays in Polynesian Ethnology*, Cambridge University Press, Cambridge, pp. 51–112, 274–275.

Wilson, J. (1799) *A Missionary Voyage to the Southern Pacific Ocean, 1796–1798, in the Ship 'Duff'*, Published privately, London.

Yuncker, T.G. (1959) *Piperaceae of Micronesia*, occasional papers, Vol. 22, Bernice P. Bishop Museum Press, Honolulu, p. 108.

5 Chemistry of Kava and Kavalactones

Iqbal Ramzan and Van Hoan Tran

Introduction

The kava shrub, *Piper methysticum* Forst., is indigenous to Oceania, where it provides the raw material for an intoxicating beverage used in feasts, rituals as well as socially at work and in home environments.

The chemical investigation of *P. methysticum* began in 1860 with the publications of Gobley (1860), O'Rorke (1860) and Cuzent (1861a,b). These authors independently reported the isolation of a neutral crystalline compound called methysticin or kavahine. It was followed by a publication from Nölting and Kopp in 1874 who reported the isolation of another neutral crystalline compound, which was later confirmed by Lewin (1886) who named this compound yangonin. Following Lewin's publication, the chemistry of the constituents of *P. methysticum* was extensively examined with the aim of identifying the active components that were responsible for the psychoactivity of kava and to characterise the structure–activity relationships of these active components. Borsche and colleagues, who published a series of fourteen papers during 1914 to 1933, contributed enormously to the elucidation of the structures of methysticin, kavain and dihydrokavain, although they failed to recognise the correct structure of naturally occurring yangonin. During this period, Winzheimer's laboratory (1908a,b) was also recognised for identifying and characterizing several active constituents of kava.

Composition and Distribution of Constituents Within the Plant

The primary bioactive compounds in kava are the kavalactones, a collective name for δ-lactones and 5,6-dihydro-δ-lactones. To date, a total of 18 kavalactones have been identified (Figure 5.1a,b). Of these, six constitute approximately 95% of the lipid extract derived from the dried roots and rhizomes, called the rootstock (Lévesque, 1985). They are kavain (also called kawain), dihydrokavain, methysticin, dihydromethysticin, yangonin, and desmethoxyyangonin. Generally, the major kavalactone content is approximately 9–12% by weight of the dried rootstock (Young *et al.*, 1966; Duve, 1981; Lebot and Lévesque, 1996) (Table 5.1), with the balance comprised of approximately 45% starch, 22% fibre, 12% water, 3% sugar, 3.5% protein, 3% minerals (Lebot and Cabalion, 1986). Typically, kavalactone concentrations are highest in the lateral roots and decrease progressively toward the aerial parts of the plant. For instance, Duve (1981) used GLC to estimate the composition of kavalactones in the root and rhizome and found that total kavalactones comprised 10.4% in the root and

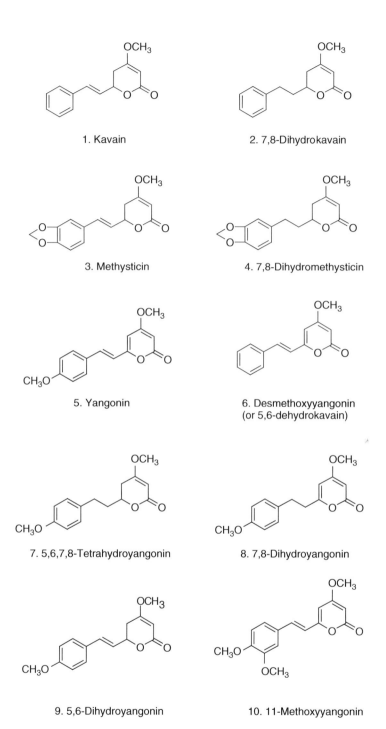

1. Kavain

2. 7,8-Dihydrokavain

3. Methysticin

4. 7,8-Dihydromethysticin

5. Yangonin

6. Desmethoxyyangonin
(or 5,6-dehydrokavain)

7. 5,6,7,8-Tetrahydroyangonin

8. 7,8-Dihydroyangonin

9. 5,6-Dihydroyangonin

10. 11-Methoxyyangonin

Figure 5.1a Chemical structures of the kavalactones isolated from the *P. methysticum* plant.

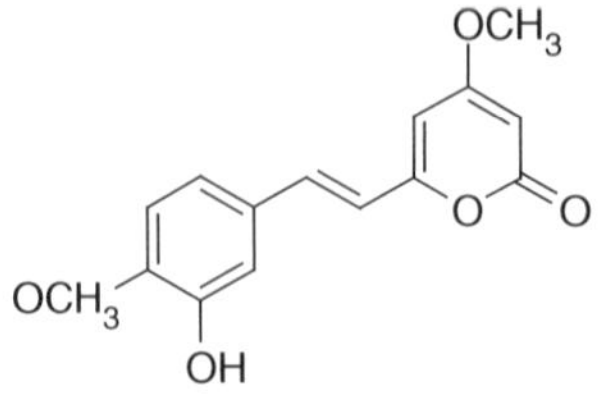

11. 11-Hydroxyyangonin

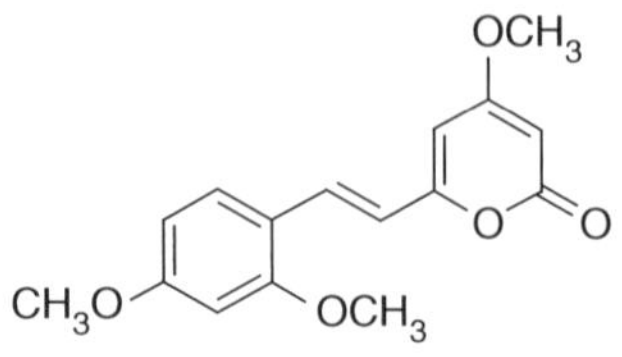

12. 10-Methoxyyangonin

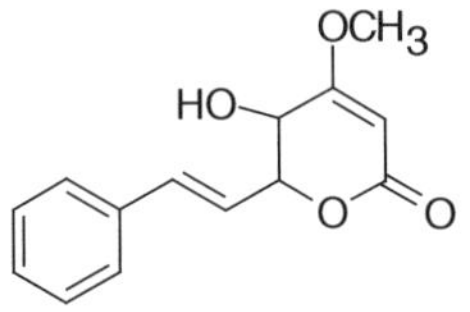

13. 5-Hydroxykavain

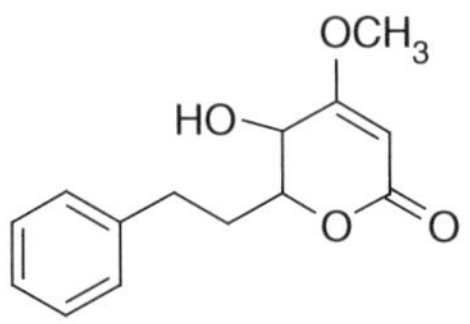

14. 5-Hydroxy-7,8-dihydrokavain

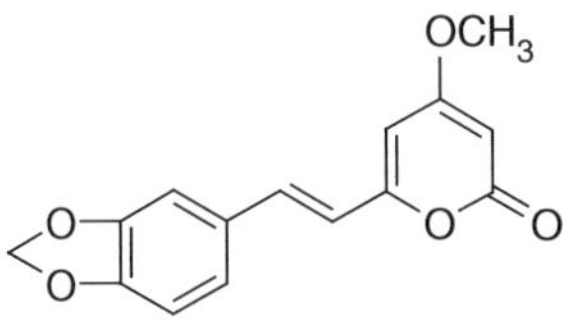

15. 5,6-Dehydromethysticin

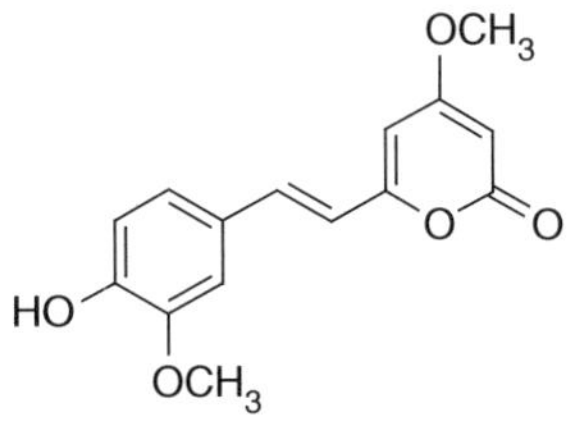

16. 11-Methoxynoryangonin

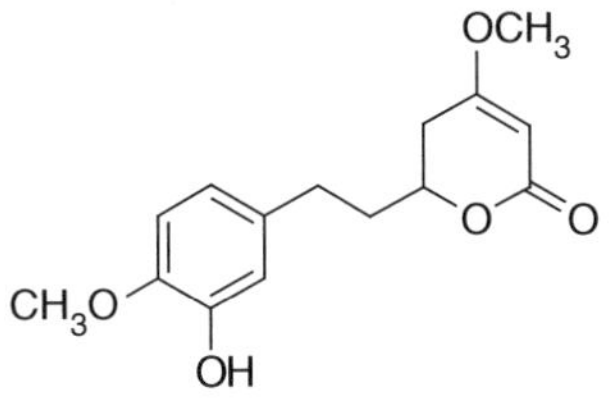

17. 11-Hydroxy-12-methoxy-
7,8-dihydrokavain

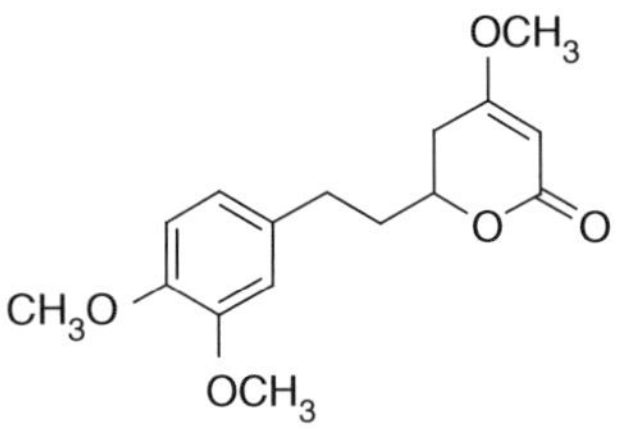

18. 11,12-Dimethoxy-7,8-
dihydrokavain

Figure 5.1b Chemical structures of the kavalactones isolated from the *P. methysticum* plant (continued).

5.2% in the rhizome. HPLC was also used to investigate more thoroughly the distribution of kavalactones in different parts of the plant, including the root, stem and the leaf. The root generally contained a majority of the unsaturated lactones such as kavain and methysticin, whereas the stem and leaf comprised mainly dihydro derivatives of kavain and methysticin (Smith *et al.*, 1984) (Table 5.2). This distribution pattern may be explained by the immediate reduction of the double bond at carbons 7 and 8 by ascorbic acid after synthesis in the leaf (Hänsel, 1968). Similarly, the stem contained a majority

Table 5.1 Major kavalactone content in weight % of dried root of *P. methysticum*

	Young et al.	*Duve*	*Lebot & Lévesque*
Kavain	2.58	1.90	2.30
Dihydrokavain	1.37	2.37	3.28
Methysticin	1.82	2.12	2.06
Dihydromethysticin	1.89	1.12	1.60
Yangonin	1.21	1.73	1.16
Desmethoxyyangonin	0.59	0.81	0.91
Total	9.46	10.05	11.31

Sources: Young *et al.* (1966): data from six samples collected in Hawaii; Duve (1981): data from six samples collected in Fiji; Lebot and Lévesque (1996): data from 121 samples collected in Vanuatu.

Table 5.2 Major kavalactone content in weight % in various parts of *P. methysticum*

	Composition of kavalactone extract (%)		
	Root	*Stem*	*Leaf*
Kavain	34.5	0.6	2.5
Dihydrokavain	17.1	23.2	69.8
Methysticin	20.8	13.9	0.8
Dihydromethysticin	5.3	59.6	22.5
Yangonin	0.8	0.8	1.2
Desmethoxyyangonin	21.6	1.8	3.0

Source: Smith (1983).

of the dihydro lactones and moderate amounts of methysticin (Smith, 1983). Yangonin was found to occur in only small amounts throughout the plant.

Kavalactone content and composition have been shown to be dependent on a number of factors, including age of the plant, plant part used as mentioned above, variety or cultivar, and geographical location and environmental conditions (Table 5.3), drying and storage conditions, extraction procedure, and analytical methods used.

Successful elucidation of the structures of kavain and its derivatives prompted chemists worldwide to search for synthetic pathways for the naturally occurring kavalactones in an effort to provide proof for the correct structures for these compounds.

Structure Elucidation of Kavalactones

In earlier times, chemical reactions, particularly alkaline hydrolysis, was the key method in the structure elucidation of the kavalactones. Among the major kavalactones, methysticin and yangonin drew much attention from chemists worldwide.

Yangonin

Yangonin was the first substance subjected to a thorough chemical examination by Borsche and colleagues (Borsche and Gerhardt, 1914; Borsche and Walter, 1927;

Table 5.3 Weight % of major constituents in total kavalactone extract from roots of *P. methysticum* from four major geographical areas of the Pacific. The number of samples analyzed is shown below the name of the country or region

	Fiji (27)	Vanuatu (67)	Polynesia* (39)	PNG/Micronesia¶ (18)
Kavain	21.03	20.30	20.29	10.88
Dihydrokavain	18.15	32.14	24.94	28.61
Methysticin	26.14	15.73	20.41	16.52
Dihydromethysticin	11.72	15.85	14.25	19.65
Yangonin	13.81	9.01	10.44	8.02
Desmethoxyyangonin	9.20	6.85	9.50	16.32

Source: Lebot and Lévesque (1989).

Notes
* constitutes Tonga (12 samples), Western Samoa (8), American Samoa (5), Wallis (3), Cook Islands (1), Tahiti and the Marquesas (3), and Hawaii (7).
¶ constitutes Papua New Guinea, Solomon Islands, Pohnpei, Palau, and Guam.

Borsche and Bodenstein, 1929), although Nölting and Kopp had already identified the substance in 1874. Yangonin is in fact a 4-methoxy-6-(*p*-methoxy-β-styryl)-α-pyrone which was not recognised by Borsche and co-workers (Borsche and Gerhardt, 1914; Borsche and Bodenstein, 1929). These authors had postulated it as a γ-pyrone, although they had correctly interpreted the structures of all other substances isolated from kava (Borsche *et al.*, 1927a,b; Borsche and Peitzsch, 1929a, 1930). Chemical behavior of yangonin (Figure 5.2) was extensively studied by Borsche's group (Borsche and Gerhardt, 1914; Borsche and Walter, 1927). Treatment of yangonin with aqueous alkali formed an acidic compound named yangonic acid, which lost a carbon dioxide molecule to form yangonol when heated. Further heat treatment of yangonic acid with alkali yielded anisaldehyde and *p*-methoxycinnamic acid. Borsche, based on the ease of decarboxylation of yangonic acid to yangonol, postulated the structure for yangonic acid shown in Figure 5.2 and proposed that yangonin was an anhydride of the methyl ester of yangonic acid.

Borsche postulated yangonin as a γ-pyrone on the evidence that the compound readily underwent saponification under mild alkaline conditions, thus, according to Borsche, it contained no enol-ether linkage in the pyrone ring (Borsche and Gerhardt, 1914). Borsche's argument for the structure of yangonin is schematically outlined in Figure 5.3. In addition, Borsche also found that yangonin readily formed an oxonium salt with platinum chloride, a typical γ-pyrone compound. He provided the final proof from a synthetic sample produced from an unambiguous synthetic scheme, which involved methylation as the final step (Borsche and Bodenstein, 1929). Borsche probably isolated only one component and used it to prove the structure of the naturally occurring yangonin. Lampe and Sandrowski (1930) were, however, unable to replicate Borsche's synthetic scheme.

The problem was later clarified with the finding that methylation of styryl-6-dihydropyran-2,4-dione, an analogue of yangonolactone, by diazomethane yielded a mixture of isomeric α-pyrone and γ-pyrone compounds as shown in Figure 5.4. These compounds were separated on the basis of the difference in solubilities of their hydrochloride oxonium salts in ether. The compound which formed an ether insoluble salt

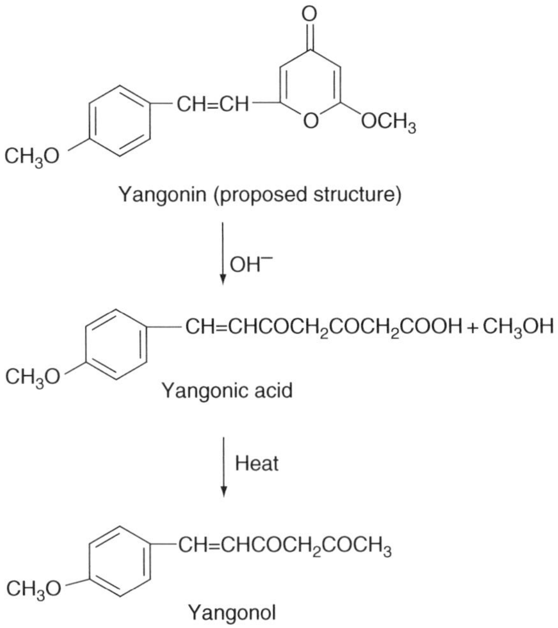

Yangonin (proposed structure)

Yangonic acid

Yangonol

Figure 5.2 Chemical reaction of yangonin under alkaline conditions and heat to yield yangonic acid and yangonol as proposed by Borsche and Walter (1927).

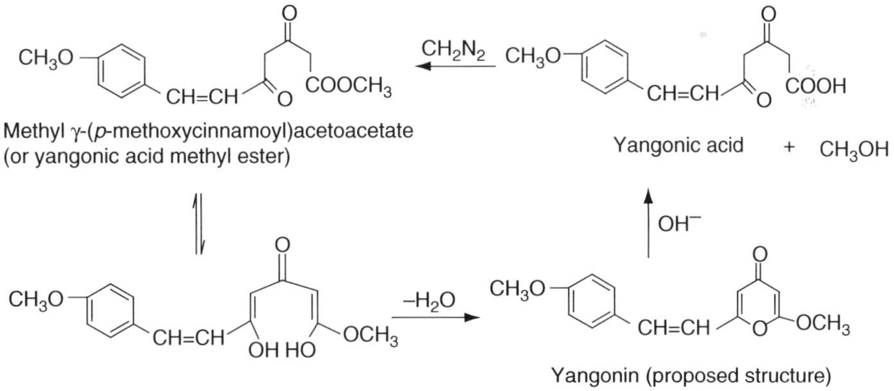

Methyl γ-(p-methoxycinnamoyl)acetoacetate (or yangonic acid methyl ester)

Yangonic acid   + CH_3OH

Yangonin (proposed structure)

Figure 5.3 Postulation of the structure for yangonin by Borsche and Gerhardt (1914).

was assigned to the γ-pyrone structure, whilst the ether soluble salt was designated as an α-pyrone (Macierewicz, 1950; Macierewicz and Janiszewska-Brozek, 1950).

Further evidence for the structure elucidation of yangonin came from the study of Chmielewska and co-workers (1958), who synthetically produced two series of isomeric pyrones, 4-methoxy-α-pyrones and 2-methoxy-γ-pyrones, the latter of which they termed pseudopyrones. Their study showed significant differences in both chemical and physical properties between the two isomeric forms. These authors were able to

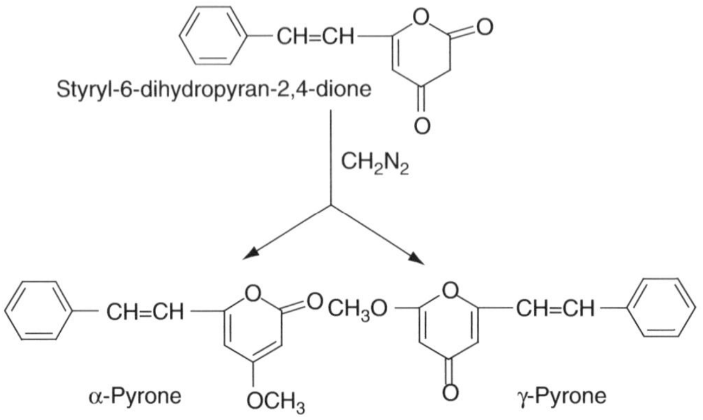

Figure 5.4 Methylation of styryl-6-dihydropyran-2,4-dione by diazomethane (Macierewicz, 1950; Macierewicz and Janiszewska-Brozek, 1950).

demonstrate differences in melting points between the two forms, where the α-pyrones, in general, had higher melting points than their corresponding pseudo-isomers. It is more significant that the ultraviolet-visible (UV) and infrared (IR) spectra of the synthetic α-pyrones were shown to be identical to that of the naturally occurring yangonin. Thus they confirmed the α-pyrone structure for naturally occurring yangonin. Herbst and co-workers later re-investigated the diazomethane methylation of 2,4-pyronones, including the synthesis of the isomers of yangonin, and confirmed Chmielewska's findings (Herbst *et al.*, 1959). Finally, Bu'Lock and Smith (1960) contributed valuable evidence confirming the α-pyrone structure of yangonin by a direct synthesis from a condensation reaction of 4-methoxy-6-methyl-α-pyrone with *p*-methoxybenzaldehyde where methylation as a final step was avoided.

Methysticin

Methysticin, a neutral compound, was first obtained in pure form by Pomerzan in 1889, following the earlier isolation by Cuzent (1861a), Gobley (1860) and O'Rorke (1860). Pomerzan successfully established its empirical formula as $C_{15}H_{14}O_5$. He also carried out hydrolysis and oxidation of the compound. Treatment of methysticin with hot alkali yielded methystic acid, which has an empirical formula of $C_{14}H_{12}O_5$. This acid was oxidized by potassium permanganate to yield 3,4-methylenedioxybenzoic acid. Methystic acid when warmed with dilute acid underwent decarboxylation to give a compound with an empirical formula of $C_{13}H_{12}O_3$, which was designated as methysticol. The easy loss of carbon dioxide from methystic acid suggested the presence of a β-keto acid which in addition to other degradation data led Pomerzan (1889) to propose, the structure for methystic acid as 7-(3',4'-methylenedioxyphenyl)-4,6-heptadienoic acid, as shown in Figure 5.5. Methysticin was considered to be the corresponding methyl ester of methystic acid. In fact, Pomerzan overlooked the presence of the methoxy group in methysticin.

It was later noted by Murayama and Shinozaki (1925) that methysticin is an optically active isomer and they argued that methystic acid was an isomerization product of methysticin. Upon acid treatment, both methystic acid and methysticin underwent decarboxylation and demethylation, respectively, yielding methysticol. Murayama and Shinozaki (1925) therefore proposed a dihydro-γ-pyrone structure for methysticin, as shown in Figure 5.6.

These authors also noted that when methysticin was treated with hot alkali, a compound named isomethysticin was obtained, which had the same empirical formula as methysticin. Borsche and co-workers (Borsche, 1927; Borsche *et al.*, 1927a) re-examined these findings and confirmed that the isomethysticin obtained by the Japanese group (Murayama and Shinozaki, 1925) was actually identical to the methystic acid obtained

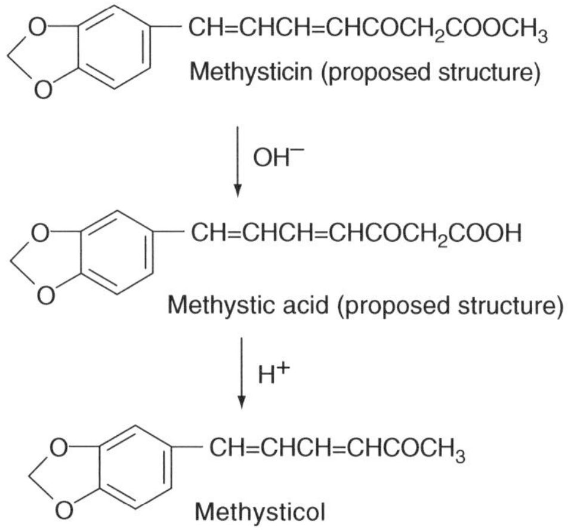

Figure 5.5 Degradation of methysticin as proposed by Pomerzan (1889).

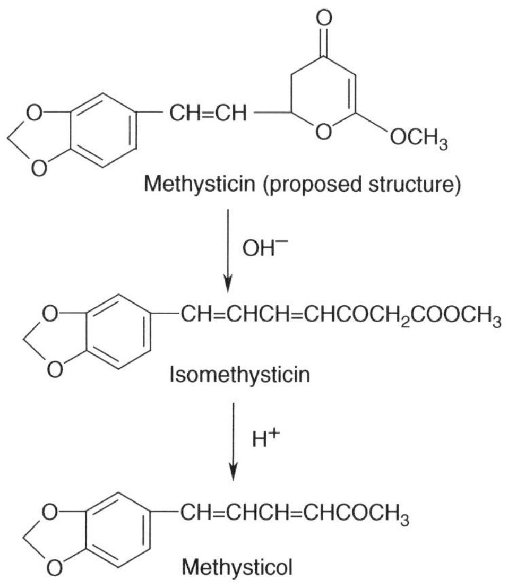

Figure 5.6 Degradation of methysticin as proposed by Murayama and Shinozaki (1925).

by Pomerzan (1889) and Winzheimer (1908a). This acidic compound was found to retain the methoxy group present in methysticin. Borsche also recognized that methystic acid was not an ester, since it could not survive the alkaline hydrolysis, but was rather a free carboxylic acid. The methoxy group was then assigned to the β-position of the carboxylic acid, which explained the easy decarboxylation and demethylation of methystic acid under acidic conditions to yield methysticol. Borsche and co-workers (Borsche *et al.*, 1927a), therefore, postulated methystic acid as 3-methoxy-7-(3′,4′-methylenedioxyphenyl)-2,4,6-heptatrienoic acid, as shown in Figure 5.7, and proposed a dihydro-α-pyrone structure for methysticin to account for these findings. The structure of methystic acid was later confirmed by synthesis (Borsche and Blount, 1930).

Further support for the structure of methysticin became available when Klohs and co-workers synthesized a racemic mixture of methysticin by the Reformatsky condensation of 3′,4′-methylenedioxycinnamaldehyde with methyl 4-bromo-3-methoxycrotonate (Klohs *et al.*, 1959a). The synthetic product exhibited identical IR and UV spectra to those of the naturally occurring methysticin. Further evidence for structural identity was obtained from treatment of both the synthetic and natural materials with alkali to yield identical products corresponding to methystic acid (Klohs *et al.*, 1959a).

7,8-Dihydromethysticin

7,8-Dihydromethysticin, a dihydro derivative of methysticin, was discovered in 1908 by Winzheimer, who named the compound as ψ-methysticin. This material was later re-examined by Borsche and Peitzsch (1929a) who found that it was a mixture of methysticin and dihydromethysticin. They further supported their claim by carrying out catalytic hydrogenation of the material to yield pure dihydromethysticin (Borsche and Peitzsch, 1929a). The compound was shown to be identical to that obtained by Goebel (1922) and Borsche (1927) from their studies on catalytic hydrogenation

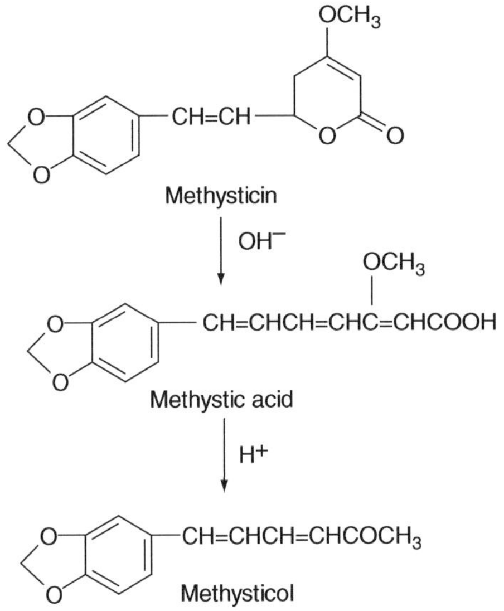

Figure 5.7 Degradation of methysticin as proposed by Borsche, Meyer and Peitzsch (1927a).

of methysticin. Klohs and co-workers finally succeeded in synthesising D,L-dihydro-methysticin in 1959 *via* hydrogenation of d,l-methysticin (Klohs *et al.*, 1959a).

Kavain and 7,8-dihydrokavain

Following the successful establishment of the structures for methysticin and dihydro-methysticin, Borsche succeeded in elucidating the structures of the subsequently isolated compounds, such as kavain and dihydrokavain (Borsche and Peitzsch, 1929a, 1930). Borsche and Peitzsch (1930) successfully established the structures of kavain and 7,8-dihydrokavain as 5,6-dihydro-α-pyrones. Borsche and Peizsch (1929b) had actually postulated the existence of kavain in the *P. methysticum* plant, before the isolation of the compound, based on the identification of kavaic acid obtained by saponifying the kava resin. Structures of kavain and dihydrokavain were later confirmed by synthesis reported by several laboratories (Fowler and Henbest, 1950; Kostermans, 1950, 1951; Viswanathan and Swaminathan, 1960; Israili and Smissman, 1976).

Desmethoxyyangonin

Of particular interest was the isolation of desmethoxyyangonin (or 5,6-dehydrokavain), one of the major kavalactone components in *P. methysticum* plant (Gottlieb and Mors, 1959a; Klohs *et al.*, 1959b). The compound was actually synthesized by Macierewicz in 1939 well before it was found to exist in the *P. methysticum* plant. In 1959, Klohs and co-workers reported the isolation of an optically inactive compound from a chloroform extract of the kava root, which they named compound A, with the empirical formula of $C_{14}H_{12}O_3$ (Klohs *et al.*, 1959b). The compound was later shown to be identical to the synthetic 5,6-dehydrokavain (Gottlieb and Mors, 1959b). It is interesting to note that this compound also occurs in other unrelated plants such as rosewoods (Gottlieb and Mors, 1958, 1959c), which belong to the *Lauraceae* family.

Other kavalactones

In recent years, several minor components have been isolated from the *P. methysticum* plant to add to the list of kavalactones, including 11-methoxyyangonin (Hänsel and Klaproth, 1966), 11-methoxynoryangonin and 5,6-dehydromethysticin (Hänsel *et al.*, 1966b). Of particular interest is that 11-methoxyyangonin and 5,6-dehydromethysticin were also identified earlier from the wood and bark of *Aniba* species (Mors *et al.*, 1962) which belongs to the Lauraceae family as mentioned above. Structures of these compounds were confirmed by synthesis (Mors *et al.*, 1962) using the method of Bu'Lock and Smith (1960). Hänsel and co-workers (Hänsel *et al.*, 1966b) were later able to reproduce structures for all three compounds in order to prove their correct structures by a synthetic method similar to that described by Bu'lock and Smith (1960).

Isolation of 11-hydroxy-12-methoxydihydrokavain and 11,12-dimethoxydihydrokavain from a methanolic extract of kava roots was also reported (Achenbach *et al.*, 1972). Physical properties of these two components, as shown in Table 5.4, were investigated in detail by these authors and their structures were confirmed by synthesis as racemic mixtures (Achenbach *et al.*, 1972).

Other kavalactones were also identified as minor components from kava rootstock, including 10-methoxyyangonin, 11-hydroxyyangonin and 11-methoxy-12-hydroxydehydrokavain

Table 5.4 Physical properties of kavalactones (1–18) and flavokavins (**FK-A**, **FK-B**, and **FK-C**). For compound numbers and abbreviations refer to Figures 5.1a, 5.1b, and 5.8; ni: not identified

Compound	Formula	Colour	Mp (°C)	α^{20}_D (solvent)	λ_{max} (nm)	Log ε_{max}	References
1	$C_{14}H_{14}O_3$	white	105–106	+105 (EtOH)	245	4.41	Borsche and Peitzsch, 1930; Hänsel et al., 1967
2	$C_{14}H_{16}O_3$	white	56–58	+30 (EtOH)	235, 260	4.04, 3.46	Borsche and Peitzsch, 1930; Hänsel et al., 1967
3	$C_{15}H_{14}O_5$	white	139–140	+95 (Acetone)	227, 267	4.39, 4.15	Klohs et al., 1959a; Hänsel et al., 1967
4	$C_{15}H_{16}O_5$	white	117–118	+20.57 (MeOH)	235, 287	4.18, 3.61	Klohs et al., 1959a; Borsche and Peitzsch, 1929a; Hänsel et al., 1967
5	$C_{15}H_{14}O_4$	yellow	153–154		361	4.39	Borsche and Bodenstein, 1929; Hänsel et al., 1967
6	$C_{14}H_{12}O_3$	yellow	138–140		231, 255, 344	4.24, 4.16, 4.42	Klohs et al., 1959a; Hänsel et al., 1967
7	$C_{15}H_{18}O_4$	white	89–90	+20 (CHCl₃)	227, 278	4.29, 3.25	Achenbach et al., 1971; Hänsel et al., 1967
8	$C_{15}H_{16}O_4$	ni	104–106		224, 278	4.10, 3.97	Duve, 1981 and references cited therein; Hänsel et al., 1967
9	$C_{15}H_{16}O_4$	ni	122–124		263	4.42	Duve, 1981 and references cited therein; Hänsel et al., 1967
10	$C_{16}H_{16}O_5$	yellow	160–161		250, 365	4.16, 4.38	Hänsel and Klaproth, 1966; Mors et al., 1962
11	$C_{15}H_{14}O_5$	ni	196–200		ni	ni	Duve, 1981 and references cited therein
12	$C_{16}H_{16}O_5$	ni	191–192		ni	ni	Duve, 1981 and references cited therein
13	$C_{14}H_{14}O_4$	ni	120–122		ni	ni	Duve, 1981 and references cited therein
14	$C_{14}H_{16}O_4$	white	92	+73 (CHCl₃)	231, 260	4.11, 2.85	Achenbach and Wittmann, 1970
15	$C_{15}H_{12}O_5$	yellow	229–230		222, 250, 361	4.41, 4.14, 4.40	Hänsel et al., 1966b, 1967
16	$C_{15}H_{14}O_5$	yellow	218–219		221, 250, 373	4.36, 4.15, 4.47	Hänsel et al., 1966b
17	$C_{15}H_{18}O_5$	white	165–167	+35 (CHCl₃)	229, 275	ni	Achenbach et al., 1972
18	$C_{16}H_{20}O_5$	white	124–125	+32 (CHCl₃)	229, 275	ni	Achenbach et al., 1972
FK-A	$C_{18}H_{18}O_5$	yellow	114–116		268, 364	3.08, 4.55	Hänsel et al., 1961
FK-B	$C_{17}H_{16}O_4$	yellow	80–82		275, 340	3.28, 4.43	Hänsel et al., 1961
FK-C	$C_{17}H_{16}O_5$	orange	195–196		245, 265, 370	3.86, 4.39, 4.58	Dutta et al., 1976

(Duve, 1981; Xian-guo *et al.*, 1997). Structures of these compounds were confirmed by synthesis by Hänsel and co-workers (Hänsel and Klaproth, 1966; Hänsel *et al.*, 1966b).

In addition, there are three hydro-derivatives of yangonin identified from the *P. methysticum* plant. These include 5,6-dihydroyangonin (Hänsel, 1968; Duve, 1981), 7,8-dihydroyangonin (Duve, 1981) and 5,6,7,8-tetrahydroyangonin (Achenbach *et al.*, 1971; Hänsel, 1968). The latter compound was actually synthesized as a racemic mixture well before the identification of its optically active enantiomer in nature by Werny and Hänsel (1963) in their investigation of structure–activity relationships of kavalactones for anti-convulsant activity. Mass spectrum of the optically active 5,6,7,8-tetrahydroyangonin was shown to be identical with that of its semi-synthetic racemic mixture which was formed by the catalytic hydrogenation of yangonin (Achenbach *et al.*, 1971). The absolute configuration of 5,6,7,8-tetrahydroyangonin was determined as (+)-enantiomer as shown in Table 5.4. Structures of the other dihydro derivatives of yangonin, however, have not as yet been fully characterized.

Hydroxylated α-pyrone derivatives, including *cis*-5-hydroxykavain (Duve, 1981) and 5-hydroxydihydrokavain (Achenbach and Wittmann, 1970), have also been isolated from *P. methysticum* as minor components. Structures of these components were later confirmed by synthesis by two independent groups (Hänsel and Schulz, 1973; Achenbach and Huth, 1974). Chemical transformation during the isolation procedure could also result in formation of 5-hydroxydihydrokavain as an artefact (Cheng *et al.*, 1988). The hydroxy group was introduced by interaction with a water molecule in an aqueous environment. It is interesting that only certain varieties of kava, particularly those from Vanuatu, appear to contain the precursor that undergoes hydroxylation (Cheng *et al.*, 1988). This finding further supports the existence of different chemotypes in the *P. methysticum*.

Alkaloids, Flavokavins and Other Components from *Piper methysticum*

There have been reports of isolation of alkaloids, such as cinnamoyl- and *m*-methoxy-cinnamoylpyrrolidines (Achenbach and Karl, 1970) and pipermethystine (Smith, 1979), flavonoids (Dutta and Ray, 1973; Dutta *et al.*, 1973, 1976; Hänsel *et al.*, 1961, 1963) including flavokavin A, B and C, ketones such as cinnamylidine-acetone and methylene 3,4-dioxycinnamylidine-acetone (Jossang and Molho, 1967), phytosterols such as stigmasterol, stigmastanol, β-sitoserol and campesterol (Jossang and Molho, 1970; Gracza and Ruff, 1986), organic acids (Achenbach and Karl, 1971) and aliphatic alcohols (Gracza and Ruff, 1986) from the *P. methysticum* plant.

Molecular Properties of Kavalactones and Alkaloids

As shown in Figure 5.1, eighteen kavalactones have been isolated so far from the *P. methysticum* plant and nine of these have been fully characterized. Some physical properties of these kavalactones are shown in Table 5.2. Six of these compounds, namely kavain, dihydrokavain, methysticin, dihydromethysticin, yangonin and desmethoxyyangonin, are present in the highest concentrations, whilst other compounds are of minor importance in the rootstock (Duve, 1981). The absolute configurations of the kavain-type compounds were determined as (*S*)-(+) enantiomers (Snatzke and Hänsel, 1968;

Beecham, 1972). Of particular interest is that none of these compounds exist as glyco-sides even though they are lactones with free hydroxyl groups on aromatic moieties. These lactones are probably deposited in the excretory cells of the *P. methysticum* plant (Hänsel, 1968). In order for this deposition to occur these substances must possess a certain degree of lipid solubility to partition into the excretory spaces. This obviously cannot happen with polar compounds, including glycosylated molecules, which do not have appropriate partition coefficients for deposition in the excretory spaces. It is also possible that the majority of the research has focused on plant resin extracts where minimal amounts of glycosides may have been present and thus escaped detection.

The basic skeleton of the lactones consists of an aromatl ring, which is linked by a two-carbon bridge to an unsaturated six-membered lactone ring (Figures 5.1a,b). A unique feature of the kavalactones is that they contain a methoxy group as part of an enol ether function, which confers significant resistance of the lactone ring toward acid and base reactions. The chemical behavior of the kavalactones was studied extensively by Borsche and co-workers during the period 1914 to 1933 in an effort to elucidate their structures.

Naturally occurring kavalactones may be classified into two structural variants which are distinguished by their degree of saturation and substitution in the aromatic moiety. All naturally occurring kavalactones invariably contain the enol functional group in the lactone ring. Interestingly, a majority of the dihydro derivatives have saturated carbons at both 5,6 and 7,8 positions. This observation supports the biosynthetic scheme first proposed by Hänsel (1968) and later confirmed by Jossang and Molho (1970). According to these authors, there are two streams in the biosynthetic pathway for kavalactones, with both pathways appearing to share the same precursor. Jossang and Molho (1970) postulated a much simpler approach than Hänsel (1968) for explaining the formation of kavalactones by two biosynthetic processes: one starts from cinnamic acid and results in yangonin-type components, whilst the other starts from the corres-ponding alcohol to yield kavain-type components (Jossang and Molho, 1970). The biosynthesis probably starts with the condensation of cinnamic acid with acetoacetic acid. The resulting molecule can then either undergo enolization followed by cyclization to form yangonin-type compounds or be subjected to reduction to form the corresponding alcohol followed by cyclization to form kavain-type products. The final products are then reduced at carbons 7 and 8 to form dihydro derivatives that occur predominantly in kavain-type compounds. In contrast, in the yangonin-type compounds, reduction of the double bond at carbons 7 and 8 causes an energetically unfavourable interruption of the long conjugated system leading to formation of less stable molecules. This reduction, however, does occur at trace levels in yangonin-type compounds, hence the formation of 7,8-dihydroyangonin and 5,6,7,8-tetrahydroyangonin.

Ultraviolet-visible and infrared spectra of kavalactones

Hänsel has provided extensive characterization of the ultraviolet-visible (UV) and infrared (IR) spectra of the kavalactones. He divided the compounds into two functional chromophores, the enolide and dienolide structures. Each of these was further divided into styryl and phenylethyl subgroups. He also used two basic molecules, methyltriace-toacid lactone (MTL) and its dihydro derivative (DHMTL) to study the UV and IR characteristics of the naturally occurring lactones (Hänsel *et al.*, 1966a, 1967; Hänsel, 1968). The IR spectra of these components are readily distinguishable on the basis of the four subgroups described above. In general, the dienolide compounds exhibit signals at 1560–1575 cm^{-1}; those that possess a styryl conjugated system exhibit an additional signal at 955–966 cm^{-1}, corresponding to the CH group in the trans-configuration at the double bond (Hänsel *et al.*, 1966a; Hänsel, 1968).

The UV spectra of the kavalactones, on the other hand, are simply divided into two structural types, yangonin- and kavain-types. Yangonin-type compounds, constituting a complete conjugated system, exhibit a bathochromic shift and display a wavelength maximum around 350 nm, which varies somewhat depending on the substitution of the auxochrome on the aromatic ring. In the kavain-type compounds, the UV spectra reflect the additive nature of the two chromophores: the aromatic moiety and the pyrone moiety. The maximum wavelength of these compounds also varies depending on the substitution on the aromatic ring and extension of the conjugated double bond at carbons 7 and 8 (Hänsel *et al.*, 1967; Hänsel, 1968).

Molecular Properties of Alkaloids

The presence of alkaloids in *P. methysticum* was first reported by Lavialle in 1889. This finding was later confirmed by Winzheimer (1908a), who successfully isolated a nitro-gen-containing liquid which yielded a crystal structure as the picrate ester. None of the subsequent investigators provided any evidence for the existence of alkaloids in the *P. methysticum* plant until 1970, when the amides, *N*-cinnamoyl pyrolidine and *m*-methoxycinnamoyl pyrolidine (Figure 5.8) were isolated from a methanolic extract of the kava root (Achenbach and Karl, 1970). Subsequently, Smith in 1979 isolated a novel pyridine alkaloid, which he named pipermethystine (Figure 5.8), from the leaves of *P. methysticum*. This alkaloid was also present in trace amounts in the roots and stems as detected using gas chromatography. Pipermethystine decomposed readily to 3-phenylpropionic acid and dihydropyridone on activated alumina during column chromatography, which had not been reported previously (Smith, 1979). A similar degradation occurred when the alkaloid was stored for several months at room temperature (Smith, 1979).

Thus the kava alkaloids contain either a cinnamoyl or phenylpropionyl moiety. One would expect that a homologous series of such alkaloids may exist in the *P. methysticum* plant, since Achenbach and Karl (1971) isolated a series of substituted cinnamic, benzoic and phenyl propionic acids. These acids would be expected to react readily with amines to form the amide alkaloids. However, such a series of alkaloids does not appear to occur in the *P. methysticum* plant, although several similar alkaloids have been isolated from other *Piper* species, such as *P. longum* which yields piplactine, piperlongumine and piperlonguminine (Chatterjee and Dutta, 1967).

Infrared spectra (IR) of these alkaloids in general exhibit a band at 1650–1690 cm^{-1} which represents the C=O bond in the amide function (Achenbach and Karl, 1970; Smith, 1979). In addition, IR spectrum of pipermethystine contains a band at 1740 cm^{-1} which represents the C=O bond in the ester function of the acetoxyl group (Smith, 1979). UV spectra of these alkaloids, however, displayed a range of wavelength maxima, attributable to the variable conjugated structures in the alkaloids. Accordingly, the cinnamoyl- and methoxycinnamoyl-pyridines exhibit bathochromic shifts to 280 and 310 nm, respectively (Achenbach and Karl, 1970). In contrast, the pipermethystine structure contains no conjugated system with the benzene ring and thus exhibits maximum UV absorption at 243 nm (Smith, 1979).

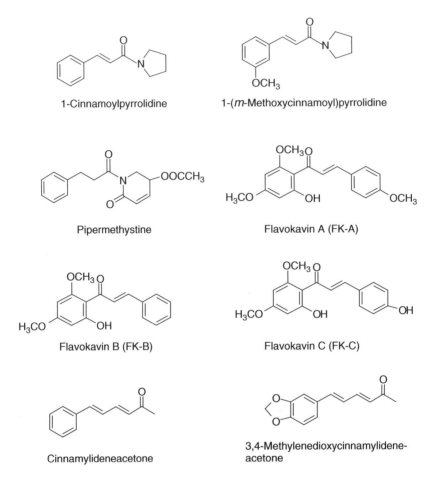

1-Cinnamoylpyrrolidine

1-(*m*-Methoxycinnamoyl)pyrrolidine

Pipermethystine

Flavokavin A (FK-A)

Flavokavin B (FK-B)

Flavokavin C (FK-C)

Cinnamylideneacetone

3,4-Methylenedioxycinnamylidene-acetone

Figure 5.8 Chemical structures of alkaloids, flavonoids and ketones isolated from the *P. methysticum* plant.

Flavokavins and Other Compounds

Three flavokavins (also known as flavokawins or flavokavains), designated A, B and C, have been identified from kava root. Structures of these compounds have been confirmed by synthesis (Hänsel *et al.*, 1963; Dutta *et al.*, 1976; Dutta and Som, 1978). The main feature of flavokavins consists of a chalcone skeleton, with each having similar substitutions on one aromatic ring as 2-hydroxy-4,6-dimethoxychalcone as shown in Figure 5.8. These compounds thus exhibit a distinct UV band at 350–370 nm (Dutta *et al.*, 1976; Hänsel *et al.*, 1963). In addition, IR spectra of flavokavins display a strong signal at 1600 cm^{-1} which represents the carbonyl group conjugated with the aromatic ring (Hänsel *et al.*, 1963; Dutta *et al.*, 1976). These flavokavins are probably synthesized, similar to kavalactones, from a mixed construction made up of one phenylpropane unit and three acetate units (Hänsel *et al.*, 1963). It is interesting to find both kavalactones and flavokavins present in the *P. methysticum* plant. Therefore it is possible that, from a biosynthetic point of view, both kavalactones and flavokavins originated from a common precursor (Hänsel *et al.*, 1963; Hänsel, 1968) and, according to Hänsel (1968), kavalactones appear to be precursors of flavonoids with one less acetate unit.

Other substances isolated from the kava resin include cinnamylidine acetone and 3,4-methylenedioxycinnamylidine acetone, as shown in Figure 5.8 (Jossang and Molho, 1967), and are probably the degradation products of kavalactones. A nitrogen-containing compound (cepharadione) has also been isolated from the kava rootstock (Jaggy and Achenbach, 1992). This type of compound is also found in other *Piper* species (Hänsel *et al.*, 1975; Hänsel and Leuschke, 1976; Desai *et al.*, 1989) and in *Cepharantha* species (Akasu *et al.*, 1974).

Analytical Techniques for the Isolation and Purification of Kavalactones

Extraction procedures basically involved refluxing dried plant materials in a *Soxhlet* extraction apparatus or simply stirring the plant material with organic solvents, either acetone, chloroform, ethanol, methanol, dichloromethane or diethyl ether. Fresh plant material, on the other hand, was normally macerated with water to obtain the juice, which was subsequently partitioned into ethyl acetate to yield the organic fraction and which, after removal of the solvent, eventually yielded the kava resin. The resin was either further fractionated directly using column chromatography or fractionated into acidic and neutral fractions followed by column chromatography to yield a more pure extract. The efficiency of the extraction procedure was dependent on the organic solvent used in the preparation of the extract, resulting in varying compositions of the kavalactones. Dichloromethane was shown to be more efficient than ethanol in the preparation of extracts for quantification of kavalactones from kava rootstock (Lopez-Avila and Benedicto, 1997). Structural modifications of the components may have also occurred during the extraction procedures, which may have introduced artefacts during extraction and analyses. Supercritical fluid extraction has been utilized recently to characterize the kavalactones. Extraction of material from kava root was performed with carbon dioxide alone and carbon dioxide with 15% ethanol as the organic modifier. Gas chromatography-mass spectroscopy (GC-MS) was used to quantify the kavalactones in the extracts. Supercritical fluid extracts displayed similar composition of kavalactones to that obtained from dichloromethane sonicated extracts (Lopez-Avila and Benedicto, 1997). In addition, there was no significant difference in the extraction efficiency of kavalactones when either pure carbon dioxide or ethanol-modified carbon dioxide was used as the extraction fluid (Ashraf-Khorassani *et al.*, 1999).

In the past, column chromatography, with acid-free alumina or silica gel, was the primary technique for producing purified extracts for subsequent analytical isolation either by thin-layer chromatography (TLC), gas liquid chromatography (GLC) or high performance liquid chromatography (HPLC). These methods together with recrystallization normally afforded a pure crystalline compound. UV spectrophotometry, infrared and mass spectrometry were the main spectroscopic techniques used in early days in the identification of functional groups and to obtain molecular fragments for structure elucidation of kavalactones. Nuclear magnetic resonance (NMR) spectroscopy appeared to play a minor role in the characterization of kava resin probably because the appropriate instrumentation was not readily available at that time. It has, however, been used widely since 1960 (Beak and Abelson, 1962; Achenbach and Wittmann, 1970; Achenbach and Regel, 1973). Revisiting the early problem of structure elucidation of naturally occurring yangonin, one would expect that NMR, if available, would have provided additional evidence to confirm the correct structure for yangonin. ^{1}H-NMR has the capability to readily distinguish protons, particularly at carbon 5 in α- and γ-pyrone structures. The proton signal at carbon 5 from γ-pyrone would display a downfield shift compared to that from α-pyrone.

TLC methods were first developed in 1966 for analytical separation of the kavalactones (Young *et al.*, 1966). TLC in combination with the colorimetric method allowed for the quantitative determination of the amount of individual kavalactones (kavain, methysticin and yangonin) present in the kava rootstock (Csupor, 1970a,b). However, when TLC proved to be inadequate, GLC methods were developed for quantitative analysis of the constituents from *P. methysticum* plant (Duve, 1981; Smith, 1983). GLC was first used in 1971 as a qualitative tool to identify kavalactones from the root (Achenbach *et al.*, 1971). GLC, however, is a destructive method that has major drawbacks since it causes decomposition of components particularly when high injection port temperatures are used. This problem of heat decomposition was overcome by the development of HPLC methods for quantitative analyses of kavalactones, first by Gracza and Ruff (1980) and then by Smith and co-workers (Smith *et al.*, 1984), who in particular successfully developed a HPLC method for quantitative analyses of kavalactones in different parts of the *P. methysticum* plant. These analytical methods all relied on the availability of analytical standards for accurate identification of the major constituents from kava resin and as such none of these methods alone provided simultaneous qualitative and quantitative analysis.

This aspect was later tackled by the Duffield group (Duffield and Lidgard, 1986; Duffield *et al.*, 1986) who successfully utilized GC coupled with MS for both qualitative and quantitative characterisation of kavalactones from kava resin. This analytical system was readily applied to the analysis of kavalactones excreted in human urine (Duffield *et al.*, 1989). The major advantage of this system was the high sensitivity that permitted the analyses to be performed on sub-microgram amounts of sample. In addition, mass spectrum of individual components from either electron impact or positive and negative ion chemical ionisation modes served as 'finger prints' for identification of their chemical structures. Improvement in such technology has made the analysis of the kavalactones even more robust. However, the disadvantage of GC (thermal decomposition) remained until the liquid chromatography-mass spectrometry (LC-MS) system was finally developed to overcome this destructive event. The remarkable development of LC interfaced with mass spectrometry (LC-MS) with the electrospray technique has played a significant role in the qualitative determination of kavalactones and other components in kava extract of the *P. methysticum* plant (Xian-guo *et al.*, 1997). This assay mode provides a subtle means of analysis, which is readily applicable to heat-labile molecules, including the kavalactones (Xian-guo *et al.*, 1997).

Separation of kavalactones was also achieved by supercritical fluid chromatography using methanol-modified carbon dioxide as the mobile phase. An optimal separation was achieved on either an amino or protein C_4 column at 125 atm and 80 °C. Semi-preparative separation of kavalactones was also obtained with two columns connected in series (Ashraf-Khorassani *et al.*, 1999). A micellar electrokinetic chromatographic method with diode-array detection has also been developed for the identification and quantitative determination of the major kavalactones from extracts of *P. methysticum* plant. Using fused-silica capillaries and a borate buffer (containing sodium taurodeoxy-cholate and β-cyclodextrin), kavain, dihydrokavain, methysticin, dihydromethysticin, yangonin and desmethoxyyangonin were successfully separated and quantified (Lechtenberg *et al.*, 1999).

Stability of Kavalactones

According to Duve and Prasad (1983), there are trends in the deterioration of the major active constituents in both dry powdered root and basal stems. Storage of the samples in screw-capped glass bottles at room temperature resulted in 26, 33 and 55% degradation of the major constituents in the roots and 24, 50 and 48% degradation in basal stems after 22, 36 and 39 months of storage, respectively. Moisture and temperature are probably the major environmental factors affecting the deterioration of dry powdered plant material. Stability of the active constituents appeared to be dependent on the chemical structure, with dihydrokavain being the least stable and methysticin the most stable (Duve and Prasad, 1983). In addition, stability improves with increasing melting point and the degree of unsaturation. These findings suggest that more polar substances are likely to be stable at room temperature. In contrast, in non-polar molecules like dihydrokavain, the pyrone ring tends to open up to form more polar acidic components which would be readily stabilized by moisture from the storage environment. The identity of the degradation products have not been established but formation of a characteristic off-odor from the samples has been described (Duve and Prasad, 1983), which probably reflects formation of the corresponding acids from the active constituents. Further studies are, however, needed before firm recommendations can be made on storage conditions for powdered kava.

Physicochemical and Pharmacokinetic Properties of the Kavalactones

The kava pyrones in general have high lipid solubility with octanol/water partition coefficients (Log P) values in the order of 3 (Rasmussen *et al.*, 1979). Thus none of these compounds were detected in the aqueous phase when they were partitioned between n-octanol and water and measured by gas–liquid chromatography. Radioactive [^{14}C]yangonin was, therefore, used to determine the partition coefficient of the compound between n-octanol and water and found to have a value of 1500 (Rasmussen *et al.*, 1979). This method not only allowed for the detection of the compound in the aqueous phase with high sensitivity but also permitted the determination of its water solubility, which was ~0.4 µg/ml (1–5 µM) at 22 °C. This extremely low aqueous solubility would be expected to have a negative impact on its dissolution and result in low and variable oral bioavailability. Urinary metabolite excretion in rats was used to estimate the extent of absorption (Rasmussen *et al.*, 1979). The 7,8-dihydro derivatives of kavain and yangonin were found to have reasonably high (~50%) bioavailability compared to the corresponding unsaturated congeners in rats. This finding indicates that the kavalactones are passively absorbed from the gastrointestinal tract. Kavain and dihydrokavain were observed to have a remarkably rapid absorption from the gastro-intestinal tract after oral administration. The peak effect in mice of these compounds, as assessed by their protection against maximal electroshock seizure, was approximately 10 minutes (Meyer, 1979). Methysticin and dihydromethysticin, in contrast, were slowly absorbed from the gastrointestinal tract after oral administration. The time of peak effect of the compounds was approximately 45 minutes. These compounds, however, appeared to be more effective than kavain and dihydrokavain in protection against electroshock seizure in mice (Meyer, 1979).

Metabolism and elimination of kavalactones in animals

Metabolism of five individual representative kavalactones were studied in rats following both oral and intraperitoneal routes at doses of 400 and 100 mg/kg, respectively. Samples collected from urine, faeces and bile were extracted with ethyl acetate, treated with a trimethylsilating agent and analysed by gas chromatography (Rasmussen *et al.*, 1979).

Dihydrokavain

Approximately 50% of the dihydrokavain from oral dose was excreted in the urine within 48 hours in the form of hydroxylated and other derivatives, including metabolites resulting from the opening of the α-pyrone ring and the hippuric acid. Six hydroxylated metabolites of dihydrokavain were identified as either mono- or dihydroxylated derivatives from which *p*-hydroxydihydrokavain was found to be the most prevalent (Rasmussen *et al.*, 1979).

Kavain

In contrast to metabolism of dihydrokavain, low amounts of metabolites were found in urine when kavain was given either intraperitoneally or orally. Its major metabolites were found to be hydroxylated kavain, dihydrokavain, and dehydrokavain and products of ring opening. Unchanged kavain, however, was excreted in large amounts in the faeces after oral dosing (Rasmussen *et al.*, 1979).

Methysticin

Similar to kavain, methysticin given orally and intraperitoneally resulted in small amounts of metabolites being excreted in the urine in 48 hours. Two major metabolites were detected and identified as *m,p*-dihydroxykavain and its dihydro derivative. These metabolites resulted from the oxidation of methylenedioxy moiety to form catechol derivatives. Of particular interest was that there were no products from ring opening of methysticin which was rather unexpected. Rasmussen *et al.* (1979) concluded that the lack of such metabolites might reflect low absorption of the compound from its site of administration. It may also reflect the high lipophilicity of methysticin favoring its demethylenation to form more polar derivatives. This phenomenon was demonstrated with the observation that the non-polar methylenedioxyphenyl compounds were extensively metabolized to the corresponding catechol derivatives, whereas polar compounds were unlikely to be metabolized *via* this pathway (Kamienski and Casida, 1970). Methysticin was also eliminated unchanged in the faeces after oral administration.

7,8-Dihydroyangonin

7,8-Dihydroyangonin, like dihydrokavain, was excreted predominantly in urine following both intraperitoneal and oral dosing. The major metabolite was identified as *p*-hydroxy-

5,6-dehydro-7,8-dihydrokavain. This metabolite resulted from 0-demethylation of the methoxy group on the aromatic ring to form a hydroxy derivative. Two other minor metabolites were also detected and identified as hydroxylated derivatives of the metabolite described above (Rasmussen *et al.*, 1979). The exact position of the hydroxyl group is yet to be determined. It was rather surprising that no evidence was obtained for the conversion of 7,8-dihydroyangonin to products of ring opening. This was in sharp contrast to that for kavain derivatives. 7,8-Dihydroyangonin is a true α-pyrone derivative and the presence of the double bond at carbon 5 and 6, extending the conjugated system, may stabilize the pyrone ring, preventing it from opening. Further investigation, however, is required to understand the metabolic differences between the kavain and yangonin compounds.

Yangonin

After both oral and intraperitoneal administration of yangonin, only small amounts of metabolites were found in urine. Metabolic transformation was similar to that for its 7,8-dihydro derivatives, in which the 0-demethylation pathway predominated (Rasmussen *et al.*, 1979). Among three metabolites detected, two had similar mass but displayed different retention times during gas–liquid chromatography. They were hypothesized to be geometrical isomers and were identified as *p*-hydroxy-5,6-dehydrokavain, in which the one with longer retention time was found to be the major metabolite. The other minor metabolite was identified as the hydroxy derivative of probably the major metabolite with unknown structure. Furthermore, negligible amounts of metabolites with all the kavalactones were detected in rat bile (Ramusssen *et al.*, 1979).

Metabolism and elimination of kavalactones in humans

Elimination of the kavalactones was also thoroughly investigated in human urine after an oral dose of a water extract of *P. methysticum* plant. In contrast to metabolism in the rat, the major fraction of the drug was excreted unchanged in the urine after overnight urinary collection (Duffield *et al.*, 1989). All six major kavalactones were detected in human urine. Metabolic transformations included the reduction of the double bond at carbons 3 and 4 to form a saturated pyrone ring system, and the demethylation of the 4-methoxy group in the α-pyrone ring. Demethylation of the 12-methoxy substituent in yangonin or alternatively hydroxylation of the aromatic ring at carbon 12 of desmethoxyyangonin was also observed. In contrast to the metabolism in rats, there were no dihydroxylated metabolites of the kavalactones, or products resulting from opening of the α-pyrone ring identified in human urine. In addition, no demethylenation of methysticin was observed in human urine (Duffield *et al.*, 1989).

Dissimilarities in the metabolism of the kavalactones between humans and rats undoubtedly demonstrate the difference in metabolic pathways between the two species. Differences may also be related to the fact that the kavalactones were given as individual components in the rat, whereas they were administered in humans as a mixture from an aqueous extract of the kava rootstock. These intriguing results with respect to the metabolism of kavalactones may also explain the observation by many early researchers that the physiological effects of the kava extract were more pronounced than with the individual lactones (Klohs *et al.*, 1959b; Steinmetz, 1960; Meyer, 1979). Therefore the lactones may be acting synergistically or may facilitate each other's transport in the gastrointestinal tract, thus enhancing their bioavailability and pharmacological activities. The extracts may also contain natural emulsifiers or carriers that may enhance the dissolution and hence the absorption processes, resulting in a higher bio-availability and more pronounced physiological effect.

Structure–activity Relationships of the Kavalactones

There was a controversial finding in early studies with respect to the effectiveness of the major kavalactones in humans since there was no correlation between their *in vivo* and *in vitro* effects. Borsche and Blount (1932) concluded that none of the substances isolated from the plant possessed any identifiable physiological activity. They thus failed to detect the important psycho-activity of the kavalactones, especially that of dihydrokavain. Although all major kavalactones can now be synthesized, these synthetic compounds appear not to produce the same physiological effects as the natural raw extract. The full efficacy of kava evidently does not reside entirely in a single active moiety but derives rather from a mixture of several kavalactones that combine to produce a synergistic physiological effect. Thus each kavalactone apparently depends on the presence of other lactones such that a more pronounced psychoactivity is observed compared to when any single isolated substance is used (Klohs *et al.*, 1959b; Meyer, 1979).

In terms of the structure–activity relationship (SAR), the psychoactive constituents basically possess a phenyl moiety linked to an α-pyrone system by a two-carbon bridge. Their potency is correlated with the lipophilicity of the molecule as a whole with dihydrokavain exhibiting the highest potency of the series. This indicates that an optimal hydrophobicity is necessary for the kavalactones to penetrate the blood-brain barrier and enter the central nervous system to exert their psycho-activity. The α-pyrone system in these compounds also plays an important role in determining their biological activity. As far as activity in animals is concerned, the lactones of the yangonin-type appear to be pharmacologically much less active at comparable doses in contrast to the kavain-type lactones (Klohs *et al.*, 1959b; Klohs, 1979). The activity of the kavain-type compounds varies with the degree of hydrogenation of the double bond at carbon 7 and substitution on the benzene ring (Meyer and Kretzschmar, 1969; Meyer, 1979). The testing method also contributes to the observed variation in the activity of the kavalac-tones. Thus kavain has the highest potency as a local anaesthetic (Meyer, 1979) and dihydrokavain as an antimycotic (Hänsel *et al.*, 1966b), whilst dihydromethysticin is the most potent potentiator of barbiturate hypnotic effect (Klohs *et al.*, 1959b; Meyer, 1962) and desmethoxyyangonin exhibits the greatest antispasmodic activity (Kretzschmar *et al.*, 1969).

Removal of the two-carbon bridge between the rings generally results in a decrease in biological activity, as assessed by the ability of the compound to protect against the convulsive effects of strychnine in animals (Klohs, 1979). This was also true when modifications were made in the substitution on the aromatic ring. Shortening or lengthening of the two-carbon bridge of dihydrokavain also decreased the fungistatic activity of the compound (Hänsel *et al.*, 1968). Extensive changes of the ethylene bridge, either by lengthening or introducing a branch in the bridge, whilst maintaining the methylenedioxy moiety of methysticin, resulted in no increase in potency of the compound as assessed by protection against the convulsive effects of strychnine in animals (Klohs, 1979). Introducing a methyl branch on the carbon adjacent to the pyrone ring of methysticin and dihydromethysticin, however, resulted in a significant increase in pentobarbital-induced sleep time in mice (Klohs, 1979). Saturation of the α-pyrone ring at carbons 5 and 6 is also a determinant of the biological activity of the kavalactones as evidenced by the anti-convulsant effects and potentiation of pentobarbital-induced sleeping time of methysticin and dihydromethysticin compared with inactive yangonin and desmethoxyyangonin (Klohs *et al.*, 1959b; Klohs, 1979). This highlights the importance of the 5,6-dihydro-α-pyrone ring to the overall pharmacological activity. Further confirmation was obtained by the complete loss of biological activity with methystic acid resulting from the opening of the lactone ring of methysticin (Klohs, 1979). In addition, saturation of the double bond at carbons 5 and 6 on the pyrone ring of yangonin resulted in a narcotic effect in the dihydro derivative in animals (Werny and Hänsel, 1963). Substitution with various groups such as methyl and phenyl groups at carbon 6 on the pyrone ring of methysticin yielded compounds with negligible pharmacological activity (Klohs, 1979). Replacement of the methoxy group on the pyrone ring of methysticin with an ethoxy group yielded an active compound that produced mild sedation in humans (Pfeiffer *et al.*, 1967).

The route of administration of kavalactones also affects the nature of the biologic activity of these compounds. The most obvious examples are yangonin and desmethoxyyangonin compounds which are relatively ineffective orally as anti-convulsants but appear to exhibit good pharmacological activity when administered parenterally (Meyer and Kretzschmar, 1969; Meyer, 1979). Substituents on the aromatic ring appeared to have the greatest effect on the potency of the kavalactones as anticonvulsants when administered intravenously. Kavain, which has no substituent on the benzene ring, was the most potent anticonvulsant, followed by methysticin, and then yangonin. However, when these compounds were administered intraperitoneally, methysticin exhibited the highest anticonvulsant activity, followed by kavain, and then yangonin (Meyer and Kretzschmar, 1969). Furthermore, the degree of saturation at carbons 7 and 8 also had a marked effect on the activity of the kavalactones as anticonvulsants when administered intraperitoneally. Compounds with a conjugated double bond at carbons 7 and 8 had the lowest anticonvulsant activity in animals (Meyer and Kretzschmar, 1969).

Yangonin and its dihydro derivative, when used in combination with other lactones, were observed to have a marked increase in potency after oral administration (Klohs *et al.*, 1959b). Recombination of the individually isolated kavalactones has also been reported to restore the pharmacological response found with the entire root extract, whilst none of the individual components appeared to have similar effects. Dihydromethysticin appeared to be the key active compound that could account for the entire plant extract potency as assessed by protection against strychnine convulsion in animals (Klohs *et al.*, 1959b).

Chemotypes

The active ingredients may be divided into the major and minor kavalactones. The former group accounts for about 96% of the whole extract (Lebot and Lévesque, 1996). As discussed in Chapter 4, some cultivars have been used for ceremonial occasions, others for medicinal purposes with particular cultivars being used to treat specific illnesses. Other cultivars were only used as a beverage and the most frequently planted cultivars were used for daily drinking (Lebot and Brunton, 1985). This traditional classification essentially reflects the physiological effect of the *P. methysticum* plant and the farmers continually select to propagate the plant with the desirable physiological effects that are thought to be correlated to a predominance of particular kavalactones. Farmers and consumers of kava are aware of this and dislike cultivars with high proportions of dihydrokavain and dihydromethysticin. On the other hand, chemotypes with high kavain content and low amounts of dihydromethysticin produce pleasant and desirable physiological effects (Lebot and Brunton, 1985).

Lebot and Cabalion (1986) carried out ethnobotanical studies on the use of kava from the Pacific countries and found that there was considerable specificity in the use of particular cultivars. Kava rootstock samples were collected from throughout the Pacific islands and analysed by HPLC. The same type of roots was systematically selected for analysis to exclude other plant material, since recent studies have shown variations in composition (and total kavalactone content) in different parts of the plant (Smith, 1979). Six major kavalactones were numbered to define the chemotypes: 1=desmethoxyyangonin (DMY); 2=dihydrokavain (DHK); 3=yangonin (Y); 4=kavain (K); 5=dihydromethysticin (DHM); and 6=methysticin. Codes were designed in decreasing order of the proportion of the lactones present thus allowing the recognition of convars, or groups of cultivars that had similar chemotypes. The first three kavalactones in the code usually represented over 70% of the total content. Over one hundred (121) cultivars of the *P. methysticum* plant originating from 51 Pacific islands, including 67 cultivars from the kava germplasm collection of Vanuatu, were analysed for the six major kavalactones. HPLC analysis data subjected to cluster analysis revealed six clusters and six distinct chemotype groups (Lebot and Lévesque, 1989, 1996). Chemotype 246531 (cluster 1) was the largest group, consisting of 32 cultivars used for daily drinking. Chemotype 426135 (cluster 2) was a group of 9 cultivars with highly pleasant, rapid but temporary physiological effects. Chemotype 264531 (cluster 3) was a group of 28 cultivars traditionally used for medicinal purposes. Chemotype 256431 (cluster 4) was a group of 26 cultivars having very pronounced and long lasting physiological effects. Chemotype 265431 (cluster 5) was a group of 16 cultivars used occasionally for ceremonial purposes and known to have very pronounced physiological effects. Chemotype 643252 (cluster 6) was a group of 10 cultivars that were always prepared from dried rather than fresh roots unlike the other chemotypes. These results demonstrated a strong correlation between the traditional use and the chemotype of a cultivar (Lebot and Lévesque, 1989, 1996).

References

Achenbach, H. and Huth, H. (1974) Synthese von Dihydrokawain-5-ol. *Tetrahedron Letters*, 1, 119–120.

Achenbach, H. and Karl, W. (1970) Uber die isolierung von zwei neuen pyrrolididen aus Rauschpfeffer (*Piper methysticum* Forst.). *Chemische Berichte*, 103, 2535–2540.

Achenbach, H. and Karl, W. (1971) Untersuchung der sauren des Rauschpfeffers (*Piper methysticum* Forst.). *Chemische Berichte*, 104, 1468–1477.

Achenbach, H., Karl, W. and Regel, W. (1972) 11-Hydroxy-12-methoxy-dihydrokawain und 11.12-dimethoxy-dihydrokawain, zwei neue kawa-lactone aus Rauschpfeffer (*Piper methysticum* Forst.). *Chemische Berichte*, 105, 2182–2187.

Achenbach, H., Karl, W. and Smith, S. (1971) Zur gaschromatograpischen trennung der kawa-lactone–(+)-5.6.7.8-tetrahydro-yangonin, ein neues kawa-lacton aus rauschpfeffers. *Chemische Berichte*, 104, 2688–2693.

Achenbach, H. and Regel, W. (1973) Inhaltssoffe des Rauschpfeffers. VI. Kernreso-nanzspektrokopische Untersuchungen an Kawalactonen. *Chemische Berichte*, **106**, 2648–2653.

Achenbach, H. and Wittmann, G. (1970) Dihydrokawain-5-ol, ein neuer alkohol aus Rauschp-feffer (*Piper methysticum* Forst.). *Tetrahedron Letters*, **37**, 3259–3262.

Akasu, M., Itokawa, H. and Fujita, M. (1974) Four new fluorescent components isolated from the callus tissue of *Stephania cepharantha*. *Tetrahedron Letters*, **41**, 3609–3612.

Ashraf-Khorassani, M., Taylor, L.T. and Martin, M. (1999) Supercritical fluid extraction of Kava lactones from Kava root and their separation via supercritical fluid chromatography. *Chromatographia*, **50**, 287–292.

Beak, P. and Abelson, H. (1962) The determination of the styryl geometry of the 6-styryl-4-methoxy-2-pyrones by proton magnetic resonance spectroscopy. *Journal of Organic Chemistry*, **27**, 3715–3716.

Beecham, A.F. (1972) The CD of α,β-unsaturated lactones. *Tetrahedron*, **28**, 5543–5554.

Borsche, W. (1927) Untersuchungen uber die bestandteile der kawawurzel. III. Uber die katalytische hydrierung des methysticins. *Chemische Berichte*, **60**, 982–984.

Borsche, W. and Blount, B.K. (1930) Untersuchungen uber die bestandteile der kawawurzel. XI. Synthese der methysticinsaure und der kawasaure. *Chemische Berichte*, **63**, 2418–2420.

Borsche, W. and Blount, B.K. (1932) Untersuchungen uber die bestandteile der kawawurzel. XII. Uber yangonalacton und triacetsaure. *Chemische Berichte*, **65**, 820–828.

Borsche, W. and Bodenstein, C.K. (1929) Untersuchungen uber die bestandteile der kawawurzel. IX. Die synthese des yangonins. *Chemische Berichte*, **62**, 2515–2523.

Borsche, W. and Gerhardt, M. (1914) Untersuchungen uber die bestandteile der kawawurzel. I. Uber yangonin. *Chemische Berichte*, **47**, 2902–2918.

Borsche, W., Meyer, C.H. and Peitzsch, W. (1927a) Untersuchungen uber die bestandteile der kawawurzel. VI. Die konstitution des methysticins. *Chemische Berichte*, **60**, 2113–2120.

Borsche, W. and Peitzsch, W. (1929a) Untersuchungen uber die bestandteile der kawawurzel. VII. Uber pseudo-methysticin. *Chemische Berichte*, **62**, 360–367.

Borsche, W. and Peitzsch, W. (1929b) Untersuchungen uber die bestandteile der kawawurzel. VIII. Uber kawasaure. *Chemische Berichte*, **62**, 368–373.

Borsche, W. and Peitzsch, W. (1930) Untersuchungen uber die bestandteile der kawawurzel. X. Uber kawain und dihydro-kawain. *Chemische Berichte*, **63**, 2414–2417.

Borsche, W., Rosenthal, W and Meyer, C.H. (1927b) Untersuchungen uber die bestandteile der kawawurzel. IV. Uber die synthese eines kawasaure-methylesters und zweier isomerer des methysticins. *Chemische Berichte*, **60**, 1135–1139.

Borsche, W. and Walter, C. (1927) Untersuchungen uber die bestandteile der kawawurzel. V. Synthese des yangonols. *Chemische Berichte*, **60**, 2112–2113.

Bu'Lock, J.D. and Smith, H.G. (1960) Pyrones. I. Methyl ethers of tautomeric hydroxypyrones and the structure of yangonin. *Journal of the Chemical Society*, 502–506.

Chatterjee, A. and Dutta, C.P. (1967) Alkaloids of *Piper longum* Linn – I. Structure and synthesis of piperlongumine and piperlonguminine. *Tetrahedron*, **23**, 1769–1781.

Cheng, D., Lidgard, R.O., Duffield, P.H., Duffield, A.M. and Brophy, J.J. (1988) Identification by methane chemical ionization gas chromatography/mass spectrometry of the products obtained by steam distillation and aqueous acid extraction of commercial Piper methysticum. *Biomedical & Environmental Mass Spectrometry*, **17**, 371–376.

Chmielewska, I., Cieslak, J., Gorzcynska, K., Knotnik, B. and Pitakowska, K. (1958) Structure de la yangonine. Etude spectrographique dans l'ultraviolet et l'infrarouge. *Tetrahedron*, **4**, 36–42.

Csupor, L. (1970a) Die quantitative Bestimmung der Kawa-Lactone in *Piper methysticum* (Forster). 1. Bestimmungsmethoden mit den Reinsubstanzen Kawain, Methysticin und Yangonin. *Archive der Pharmazie*, **303**, 193–200.

Csupor, L. (1970b) Die quantitative Bestimmung der Kawa-Lactone in *Piper methysticum* (Forster). 2. Die Bestimmung von Kawain, Methysticin und Yangonin in Rhizome Kawa-Kawa. *Pharmazie*, **25**, 197–198.

Cuzent, G. (1861a) Composition chimique de la kavahine. *Comptes Rendus Hebdomadaires des Seances de L'Academie des Sciences*, **52**, 205–206.

Cuzent, G. (1861b) De la racine de kawa. *Journal de Pharmacie et de Chimie*, **39**, 202–204.

Desai, S.J., Chaturvedi, R.N., Badheka, L.P. and Mulchandani, N.B. (1989) Aristolactams and 4,5-dioxoaporphines from Indian *Piper* species. *Indian Journal of Chemistry, Section B*, **28B**, 775–777.

Duffield, A.M., Jamieson, D.D., Lidgard, R.O., Duffield, P.H. and Bourne, D.J. (1989) Identification of some human urinary metabolites of the intoxicating beverage kava. *Journal of Chromatography*, **475**, 273–281.

Duffield, A.M. and Lidgard, R.O. (1986) Analysis of kava resin by gas chromatography and electron impact and methane negative ion chemical ionization mass spectrometry. New trace constituents of kava resin. *Biomedical & Environmental Mass Spectrometry*, **13**, 621–626.

Duffield, A.M., Lidgard, R.O. and Low, G.K.C. (1986) Analysis of the constituents of *Piper methysticum* by gas chromatography methane chemical ionization mass spectrometry. New constituents of kava resin. *Biomedical & Environmental Mass Spectrometry*, **13**, 305–313.

Dutta, C.P. and Ray, L.P.K. (1973) Further studies on the structure of flavokawain-C. A new chalcone isolated from *Piper methysticum*. *Indian Science Congress Association Proceedings*, **60**, 121–122.

Dutta, C.P., Ray, L.P.K., Chatterjee, A. and Roy, D.N. (1973) Constitution of flavokawain-C. *Indian Journal of Chemistry*, **11**, 509–510.

Dutta, C.P., Ray, L.P.K., Chatterjee, A. and Roy, D.N. (1976) Studies on the genus *Piper*. V. Chemical investigation of *Piper methysticum* Forst. (Piperaceae). Structure and synthesis of flavokawain-C. *Journal of Indian Chemical Society*, **53**, 1194–1197.

Dutta, C.P. and Som, U.K. (1978). Studies on the genus *Piper* – VIII. Further studies on the roots of *Piper methysticum* Forst. *Journal of Indian Chemical Society*, **55**, 932–934.

Duve, R.N. (1981) Gas–liquid chromatographic determination of major constituents of *Piper methysticum. Analyst*, **106**, 160–165.

Duve, R.N. and Prasad, J. (1983) Changes in chemical composition of "yaqona" (*Piper methysticum*) with time. *Fiji Agriculture Journal*, **45**, 45–50.

Fowler, E.M.F. and Henbest, H.B. (1950) Researches on acetylenic compounds. XXV. Synthesis of (±) kawain. *Journal of Chemical Society*, 3642–3645.

Gobley, M. (1860) Recherches chimiques sur la racine de kawa. *Journal de Pharmacie et de Chimie*, **37**, 19–23.

Goebel, H. (1922) Zur katalytischen hydrierung des Methysticins. *Berichte der Deutschen Pharmazeutischen Gessellschaft*, **32**, 115–124.

Gottlieb, O.R. and Mors, W.B. (1958) Isolamento de 4-Metoxi-paracotonia e 5,6-Dihidrocavaina da *Aniba firmula*. *Anais da Academia Brasileira de Ciências*, **30**, 527–528.

Gottlieb, O.R. and Mors, W.B. (1959a) Sobre a Ocorrencia da 5,6-Dehidrocavaina na Raiz de Cava. *Anais da Academia Brasileira de Ciências*, **31**, 407–409.

Gottlieb, O.R. and Mors, W.B. (1959b) Identity of compound A from kava root with 5,6-dehydrokawain. *Journal of Organic Chemistry*, **24**, 1614–1615.

Gottlieb, O.R. and Mors, W.B. (1959c) The chemistry of rosewood. III. Isolation of 5,6-dehydrokawain and 4-methoxy-paracotoin from *Aniba firmula* Mez. *Journal of Organic Chemistry*, **24**, 17–18.

Gracza, L. and Ruff, P. (1980) Einfache Methode zur Trennung und quantitativen Bestimmung von Kawa-Laktonen durch Hochleistungs-Flussigkeits-Chromatographie. *Journal of Chromatography*, **193**, 486–490.

Gracza, L. and Ruff, P. (1986) Uber die hoheren Alkohole von *Piperis methystici* rhizoma: Aliphatic and alicyclic alcohols of *Piperis methystici* rhizoma. *Archive der Pharmazie*, **319**, 475–477.

Hänsel, R. (1968) Characterization and physiological activity of some kawa constituents. *Pacific Science*, **22**, 293–313.

Hänsel, R., Bahr, P. and Elich, J. (1961). Isolierung und Charakterisierung von zwei bisher unbekannten Farbstoffen des Kawa-Rhizoms. *Archive der Pharmazie*, **294**, 739–743.

Hänsel, R. and Klaproth, L. (1966) Isolierung von 11-methoxy-yangonin aus der kawawurzel. *Archive der Pharmazie*, **299**, 503–506.

Hänsel, R., Langhammer, L. and Rimpler, H. (1967) Analytische studien an kava-laktonen: UV-absorptiometrische untersuchengen. *Archive der Pharmazie*, **300**, 157–168.

Hänsel, R. and Leuschke, A. (1976) Ein Aporphinalkaloid aus *Piper sanctum*. *Phytochemistry*, **15**, 1323.

Hänsel, R., Leuschke, A. and Gomez-Pompa, A. (1975) Aporphine-Type Alkaloids from *Piper auritum*. *Lloydia*, **38**, 529–530.

Hänsel, R., Ranft, G. and Bahr, P. (1963) Zwei Chalkonpigmente aus *Piper methysticum* Forst. 4. Mitt. Zur Frage der Biosynthese der Kawalaktone. *Zeitschrift für Naturforschung*, **18b**, 370–373.

Hänsel, R., Rimpler, H. and Langhammer, L. (1966a) IR-Spektren der α-pyrone vom yangonin-und kawain-type und synthese von 4-methoxy-5,6-dihydro-6-methyl-pyron-2 als modellsubstanz. *Zeitschrift für Analytische Chemie*, **218**, 346–353.

Hänsel, R., Sauer, H. and Rimpler, H. (1966b) 11-Methoxy-nor-yangonin aus einer botanisch nicht beschriebenen Piperart Neu-Guineas. *Archive der Pharmazie*, **299**, 507–512.

Hänsel, R. and Schulz, J. (1973) Synthese von racem 5,6-*cis*- und *trans*-kawain-5-ol. *Chemische Berichte*, **106**, 570–575.

Hänsel, R., Weiss, D. and Schmidt, B. (1968). Kawalaktone: Kettenlange und fungistatische Wirkung. *Archive der Pharmazie*, **301**, 369–373.

Herbst, D., Mors, W.B., Gottlieb, O.R. and Djerassi, C. (1959) Naturally occurring oxygen heterocyclics. IV. The methylation of pyronones. *Journal of American Chemical Society*, **81**, 2427–2430.

Israili, Z.H. and Smissman, E.E. (1976) Synthesis of kavain, dihydrokavain and analogues. *Journal of Organic Chemistry*, **41**, 4070–4074.

Jaggy, H. and Achenbach, H. (1992) Cepharadione A from *Piper methysticum*. *Planta Medica*, **58**, 111.

Jossang, P. and Molho, D. (1967) Chromatographie sur couches epaisses non liees des constituants du rhizome de *Piper methysticum*: Isolement de deux nouvelles cetones, cinnamalacetone et methylene dioxy-3,4 cinnamalacetone. *Journal of Chromatography*, **31**, 375–383.

Jossang, P. and Molho, D. (1970) Etude des constituants des feuilles de *Piper methysticum* Forst. *Bulletin du Museum National D'Histoire Naturelle*, **2**, 440–447.

Kamienski, F.X. and Casida, J.E. (1970) Importance of demethylation in the metabolism *in vivo* and *in vitro* of methylenedioxyphenyl synergists and related compounds in mammals. *Biochemical Pharmacology*, **19**, 91–112.

Klohs, M.W. (1979) Chemistry of Kava. In D.H. Efron, B. Holmstedt and N.S. Kline (eds), *Ethnopharmacologic Search for Psychoactive Drugs*, Raven Press, New York, pp. 126–132.

Klohs, M.W., Keller, F. Williams, R.E. (1959a) *Piper methysticum* Forst. II. The synthesis of d,l-methysticin and d,l-dihydromethysticin. *Journal of Organic Chemistry*, **24**, 1829–1830.

Klohs, M.W., Keller, F., Williams, R.E., Toekes, M.I. and Cronheim, G.E. (1959b) A chemical and pharmacological investigation of *Piper methysticum* Forst. *Journal of Medicinal and Pharmaceutical Chemistry*, **1**, 95–103.

Kostermans, D.G.F.R. (1950) Synthesis of kawain. *Nature*, **166**, 788–789.

Kostermans, D.G.F.R. (1951) The synthesis of kawain. *Recueil des Travauz Chimiques*, **70**, 79–82.

Kretzschmar, R., Meyer, H.J., Teschendorf, H.J. and Zoellner, B. (1969) Spasmolytische Wirksamkeit von Aryl-Substituierten a-Pyronen und Wassrigen Extrakten aus *Piper methysticum* Forst. *Archives Internationales de Pharmacodynamie et de Thérapie*, **180**, 475–491.

Lampe, V. and Sandrowski, S. (1930) Etudes sur la synthese de la methysticine. *Bulletin Societié Chimique der France*, **47**, 469–479.

Lavialle, M. (1889) La kavaine. *L' Union Pharmaceutique*, **30**, 5.

Lebot, V. and Brunton, R. (1985) Traditional Plants as Cash Crops: A Survey of Kava (*Piper methysticum* Forster) in Vanuatu. *Report Paper – Department of Agriculture*, 7pp.

Lebot, V. and Cabalion, P. (1986) Les Kavas de Vanuatu (cultivars de *Piper methysticum* Forst.). *Travaux et Documents de l'ORSTOM*, CNRS, Paris, **205**, 1–260.

Lebot, V. and Lévesque, J. (1989) The origin and distribution of kava (*Piper methysticum* Forst. F., Piperaceae): a phytochemical approach. *Allertonia*, 5, 223–281.

Lebot, V. and Lévesque, J. (1996) Genetic control of kavalactone chemotypes in *Piper methysticum* cultivars. *Phytochemistry*, 43, 397–403.

Lechtenberg, M., Quandt, B., Kohlenberg, F.-J. and Nahrstedt, A. (1999) Qualitative and quantitative micellar electrokinetic chromatography of kavalactones from dry extracts of *Piper methysticum* Forst. and commercial drugs. *Journal of Chromatography* A, 848, 457–464.

Lévesque, J. (1985) Rapport préliminaire sur l'étude chimique d'échantillons de Kava (*Piper methysticum*) sélectionnés par La Station d'Agriculture de Tagabé, République de Vanuatu. Université de Poitiers, Laboratoire de Pharmacognosie, 41pp.

Lewin, L. (1886) Uber *Piper methysticum* (kawa-kawa). Monograph, Medical Society, August Hirschwald, Berlin, 60pp.

Lopez-Avila, V. and Benedicto, J. (1997) Supercritical fluid extraction of kava lactones from *Piper methysticum* (kava) herb. *HRC-Journal of High Resolution Chromatography*, 20, 555–559.

Macierewicz, Z. (1950) Synthesis of the lactone of the mother substance of yangonin. *Roczniki Chemique*, 24, 144–166.

Macierewicz, Z. and Janiszewska-Brozek, S. (1950) Structure of α-substituted-α-γ-pyronones. *Roczniki Chemique*, 24, 167–176.

Meyer, H.J. (1962) Pharmacologie der wirksamen prinzipien des kawa-rhizoms (*Piper methysticum*, Forst). *Archives Internationales de Pharmacodynamie*, 138, 505–536.

Meyer, H.J. (1979) Pharmacology of kava. In D.H. Efron, B. Holmstedt and N.S. Kline (eds), *Ethnopharmacologic Search for Psychoactive Drugs*, Raven Press, New York, pp. 133–140.

Meyer, H.J. and Kretzschmar, R. (1969) Untersuchungen über Beziehungen zwischen Molekularstruktur und pharmakologischer Wirkung C_6-arylsubstituierter 4-Methoxy-α-pyrone vom Typ der Kawa-Pyrone. *Arzneimittelforschung*, 19, 617–623.

Mors, W.B., Magalhaes, M.T., Lima, O.R., Bittencourt, A.M. and Gottlieb, O.R. (1962) A quimica do genero *Aniba*. XI. Isolamento e sintese de 11-metoxi-iangonia e de 5,6-dehidrometisticina. *Anais da Associacao Brasileira de Quimica*, 21, 7–12.

Murayama, Y. and Shinozaki, K. (1925) Constituents of the kawa kawa. II. Constitution of methysticins. *Journal of Pharmaceutical Society of Japan* (*Yakugaku Zasshi*), 520, 526–529.

Nölting, E. and Kopp, A. (1874) Sur la racine de kawa. *Moniteur Scientifique*, 920–923.

O'Rorke, M. (1860) *Comptes Rendus Hebdomadaires des Seances de L'Academie des Sciences*, 50, 598.

Pfeiffer, C.C., Murphree, H.B. and Goldstein, L. (1967) Effect of kava in normal subjects and patients. In D.H. Efron, B. Holmstedt and N.S. Kline (eds), *Ethnopharmacologic Search for Psychoactive Drugs*, Raven Press, New York, pp. 155–161.

Pomerzan, C. (1889) Uber das methysticin. *Monastshefte fur Chemie*, 10, 783–793.

Rasmussen, A.K., Scheline, R.R., Solheim, E. and Hänsel, R. (1979) Metabolism of some kava pyrones in the rat. *Xenobiotica*, 9, 1–16.

Smith, R.M. (1979) Pipermethystine, a novel pyrone alkaloid from *Piper methysticum*. *Tetrahedron*, 35, 437–439.

Smith, R.M. (1983) Kava lactones in *Piper methysticum* from Fiji. *Phytochemistry*, 22, 1055–1056.

Smith, R.M., Thakrar, H., Arowolo, T.A. and Shafi, A.A. (1984) High-performance liquid chromatography of kava lactones from *Piper methysticum*. *Journal of Chromatography*, 283, 303–308.

Snatzke, G. and Hänsel, R. (1968) Die Absolutkonfiguration der Kawa-Lactone. *Tetrahedron Letters*, 15, 1797–1799.

Steinmetz, E.F. (1960) *Piper methysticum* (kava). *Famous Drug Plant of the South Sea Islands*. Amsterdam, 46pp.

Viswanathan, K. and Swaminathan, S. (1960) d,l-Marindinin (dihydrokawain) and some related 6-aryl-5,6-dihydro-4-methoxy-2-pyrones. *Proceedings of the Indian Academy of Science*, 52, 63–68.

Werny, F. and Hänsel, R. (1963) Die Hydrierung von 6-Styryl-α-Pyronen zu Wirkstoffen vom Typus der Kawa-Laktone (aus *Piper methysticum*). *Naturwissenschaften*, 50, 355.

Winzheimer, E. (1908a) Beitrage zur Kenntnis der Kawawurzel. *Archive der Pharmazie*, 246, 338–365.

Winzheimer, E. (1908b) Über die Identitat von Methysticol und Piperonylenaceton. *Chemische Berichte*, 41, 2377–2383.

Xian-guo, H., Long-ze, L. and Li-zhi, L. (1997) Electrospray high performance liquid chromatography-mass spectrometry in phytochemical analysis of kava (*Piper methysticum*) extract. *Planta Medica*, 63, 70–74.

Young, R.L., Hylin, J.W., Plucknett, D.L., Kawano, Y. and Nakayama, R.T. (1966). Analysis for kawa pyrones in extracts of *Piper methysticum*. *Phytochemistry*, 5, 795–798.

6 Pharmacology and Toxicology of Kava and Kavalactones

Yadhu N. Singh

Introduction

Although methysticin had been isolated in 1860–61, no pharmacological evaluation of the kavalactones was available until Lewin published his admirable monograph (Lewin, 1886). However, since only limited quantities of methysticin and yangonin were at his disposal, his data must now be considered to be only of historical importance. Nonetheless, they are worth mentioning. Methysticin was found to be inactive when injected intraperitoneally in doses of up to 2 g in both warm- and cold-blooded animals. Yangonin, available in even smaller quantities, was tested in only two frogs in oral doses of 0.05 g with no observable effects.

The bulk of Lewin's experiment was carried out on the resin remaining after the crystallization of methysticin and yangonin. It produced paralysis in frogs and exhibited a local anesthetic action. In experiments with a bat, a sparrow, and a pigeon, it caused the loss of use of the wings and the animals appeared to be deeply sedated. Subcutaneous administration of the material in cats resulted in a deep sleep with obvious local anesthetic activity, but when given orally, only salivation and vomiting were noted.

Early studies

Following the extensive chemical studies done in his laboratory over a period of over 20 years, Borsche came to the conclusion that none of the kavalactones known at that time (i.e., methysticin, dihydromethysticin, yangonin, dihydrokavain, and kavain) possessed the biological activities reputed to be present in the crude preparation (Borsche and Blount, 1933). The possibility that the active principle(s) might be present in the unsaponifiable fraction could not be substantiated, as the solubility characteristics of the fraction did not allow for biological testing. In a pharmacological investigation carried out a few years earlier, Schübel (1924) found the kava resin to have a weak narcotic action, to paralyze sensory nerves and to first stimulate, then paralyze smooth muscles. The hydrolysis products of this resin also showed similar actions. The local anesthetic action was attributed to compounds containing benzoic and cinnamic acid residues. In experiments in the isolated frog heart, Schübel showed that incubation of the kava root with human saliva increased the potency of kava extract. He attributed the increase in activity to the enzymatic breakdown of starch in the root, which in turn led to a more efficient extraction of the active material. However, Schübel was unable to demonstrate any pharmacological activity when the pure compounds yangonin and methysticin were administered to rabbits, pigeons, or frogs.

Van Veen (1938) employed pigeons, monkeys, and rice birds to follow the active principles of kava in his isolation procedure. Preliminary results indicated that rice birds were overly sensitive to the crude extracts and monkeys too resistant. Pigeons were thereafter used for routine assays. Eight to 15 minutes after administration of the extract, the pigeons became sleepy and ataxic; a deep sleep then set in lasting from 2 to 10 hours. The birds appeared to be fully recovered upon awakening. Monkeys required three to five times the dose used in pigeons. An effective dose caused initial loss of limb control, followed by sleep within 15–30 minutes which lasted for 15 hours or longer. Van Veen found that purified fractions gave a maximal effect when administered in an oil or lecithin-water emulsion and consequently proposed that chewing the root and admixing saliva only served to bring about emulsification and thus promote activity.

Van Veen succeeded in isolating an active fraction from which he reported a crystalline material and which he called *marindinin* after the Marind-Anim district in New Guinea, now known as Kolepom. He subsequently demonstrated that marindinin was a slightly impure form of dihydrokavain, a compound found by Borsche to be physiologically inactive. Van Veen also tested the purified dihydrokavain and showed that the pharmacological activity he had earlier demonstrated was indeed due to this refined material and not to the impurity.

Work in several laboratories subsequently confirmed the activities of the kavalactones. Hänsel and Beiersdorff (1959) showed that dihydrokavain and dihydromethysticin both appeared to be active in causing sleep in white mice and white rats when administered orally by a stomach tube as an emulsion. Meyer *et al*. (1960) reported that dihydrokavain and dihydromethysticin had sedative activity when administered intraperitoneally or orally to mice, rats, rabbits, and cats. Higher doses led to a marked ataxic phase followed by loss of the righting reflex. When administered to mice as peanut oil solutions, both dihydrokavain and dihydromethysticin produced sedation, hypothermia, and a corresponding reduction in total oxygen consumption. In anesthetized rabbits, blood pressure was only slightly reduced (Meyer, 1962). These findings, however, could not be replicated by Keller and Klohs (1963) and are reminiscent of the contradictory evidence of Borsche and Van Veen mentioned earlier.

Klohs *et al*. (1959) studied the effects of the ground root of kava (a chloroform extract obtained therefrom and several of its crystalline constituents) on the central nervous system as determined by their ability to antagonize clonic strychnine convulsions and death in mice, to cause fall-out in roller cage experiments and to potentiate sodium pentobarbital-induced sleeping time. The crude extract, methysticin, and dihydromethysticin were particularly effective in affording protection against the lethal effects of strychnine, while yangonin and dihydroyangonin were practically without effect. Kavain and dihydrokavain were only moderately effective. All of the compounds increased pentobarbital-induced sleeping time with dihydromethysticin being the most potent. Using fall-out from revolving (roller) cages as an index, none of the crystalline compounds had significant activity. This was in sharp contrast to the ground root and the crude extract. On the basis of these results, Klohs *et al*. (1959) proposed the presence of a synergistic action for the individual compounds when administered in combination. An indication of a synergistic effect was also found by testing a mixture of kavain, dihydrokavain, methysticin, dihydromethysticin, yangonin, and dihydroyangonin against strychnine convulsions and death. The amounts of the compounds tested were in the ratio in which they were isolated from the crude extract. The mixture showed potency similar to that of dihydromethysticin. Since this agent represented only about 5% of the mixture, and since the other constituents were less potent or inactive, a synergistic effect of the mixture appeared the most likely explanation. In agreement with Klohs *et al.* (1959), Meyer (1979) reported that the activity of yangonin and desmethoxyyangonin (administered intraperitoneally, ip) in preventing mice from maximal electroshock seizure was markedly increased when given in combination with the other kava constituents.

Frater (1958), working in Fiji with medical students (ethnic background not indicated but probably comprising Pacific islanders and Indo-Fijians), also observed the effects of kava on the nervous system in human subjects. Following the consumption of six pints of an infusion (composition not given) over a 2 hour period, the subjects looked sleepy, their eyes were slightly bloodshot and definitely watery, with the pupils enlarged and reacting only slowly to light. Speech was only slightly affected. The subjects were able to walk in a straight line and could still run up the stairs two at a time. The local anesthetic action of the lactones originally observed by Lewin (1886), Schübel (1924), and others early in the twentieth century was also reinvestigated. Frater (1958) showed that a thin paste of kava powder, when applied to the mucous membrane of the lip, produced a slight burning sensation and a feeling of numbness. With a pinprick test there was some impairment of feeling as compared with the rest of the lip. When some root was chewed for 15 minutes, however, the degree of anesthesia was greater leading him to conclude that there was a definite local anesthetic effect.

Pharmacodynamic Studies

Anesthesia and sedation

The pentobarbital-induced sleeping time in female Carworth mice was prolonged by 340% after oral (po) administration of 160 mg/kg bodyweight of a solvent-free chloroform extract of kava root (Klohs *et al.*, 1959). In comparison, purified single lactones in the same dose were less effective (150–235%), except for dihydromethysticin for which 60 mg/kg increased sleeping time by 413%. On the other hand, Meyer (1966) found that methysticin (minimal effective dosage was 20 mg/kg in mice) was the most effective, followed by kavain, dihydrokavain, and yangonin. A prolongation of pentobarbital sodium-induced (50 mg/kg) sleeping time in mice by pretreatment with kava resin (120 mg/kg) but not with an aqueous extract of kava (250 mg/kg) has also been reported by Duffield and Jamieson (1988). Hexobarbital sodium (200 mg/kg ip) produced a maximal period of lateral recumbent position of about three hours. After the animals had been pre-treated with dihydromethysticin (40 mg/kg ip), the same effect was achieved with 70 mg/kg of the barbiturate. With the use of an EEG, it was shown that kavalactones prolong and deepen anesthesia and consequently bring about potentiation and prolongation of anesthesia (Meyer, 1962). However, in a more recent study (Holm *et al.*, 1991), the percentage duration of active wakefulness was significantly shortened ($P < 0.05$) by both (±)-kavain, the synthetic racemate of the natural kavain, and pentobarbital, as compared to placebo. There was likewise a significant prolongation ($P < 0.02$) of synchronized sleep with (±)-kavain, pentobarbital, and a combination of these two compounds. However, a potentiation of drug effects failed to occur.

Analgesia and local anesthetic effects

The analgesic actions of the kava constituents dihydrokavain and dihydromethysticin were investigated utilizing the Gross modification of the Hardy, Wolff, and Goodell radiant heat method (Brüggemann and Meyer, 1963). Both kavalactones in doses of 100–140 mg/kg ip had analgesic activity as indicated by an increase in reaction time, with dihydromethysticin producing about a 1.3 times higher level of anesthesia than dihydrokavain and acetylsalicylic acid (200 mg/kg), being almost equipotent to aminopyrine (100 mg/kg) and being inferior to morphine (2.5 mg/kg). There was active synergism with the simultaneous administration of individual lactones with aminopyrine or acetylsalicylic acid, while caffeine diminished the duration of analgesic activity without affecting the peak response.

In another study, most of the kavalactones inhibited frog heart contraction (Meyer and May, 1964). These actions were compared with those of cocaine which showed a similar protection against ventricular fibrillation through its local anesthetic effectiveness. Similar effects were noted later by Meyer (1979).

Some of the analgesia properties of the kavalactones were deduced from their antinociceptive activity using various methods in mice. In the tail immersion test, the mouse tail was immersed to a depth of about 2 cm in water at 48 °C and the prolongation of time from immersion to withdrawal was considered a measure of the degree of analgesic activity. Kava resin (150 mg/kg ip) and aqueous kava extract (250 mg/kg ip) prolonged reaction time from 19.7 to 49.7 seconds ($P < 0.001$) and 10.1 to 18.8 seconds ($P < 0.025$), respectively. The peak analgesia was reached about 10 minutes after injection and persisted for 80–90 minutes (Jamieson *et al.*, 1989). Of the purified lactones tested, kavain, dihydrokavain, methysticin, and dihydromethysticin had potent analgesic properties. The peak effect was similar for the four compounds, but the time course of action differed markedly. The action of dihydrokavain was most rapid but short-lived (20–30 minutes), that of kavain a little more prolonged, while the actions of methysticin and dihydromethysticin were more persistent (about 4 hours). The yangonins, on the other hand, had negligible or no effect, even up to a dosage of 1 g/kg ip (Jamieson *et al.*, 1989; Jamieson and Duffield, 1990a,b). In the hot plate test, the time to elicit a flick by a hind limb held against a hot plate heated to 56 °C was considered the reaction time to the noxious stimulus. The aqueous kava extract (250 mg/kg) significantly prolonged the reaction time to the hot plate from 10.3 to 13.4 seconds ($P < 0.05$).

The writhing test was used to determine chemical-induced visceral pain sensitivity. Mice were injected with acetic acid (0.1 ml/kg of 0.8% acetic acid) and the number of writhes with or without pretreatment with kava resin (200 mg/kg po) or aqueous kava extract (200 mg/kg ip) was recorded. The number of pain-dependant reactions per minute was significantly ($P < 0.001$) reduced, from 22.9 to 11.3 with kava resin and from 22.7 to 3.2 with aqueous kava, indicating a pronounced analgesic effect with both preparations. The authors also raised the possibility that the muscle-relaxant and sedative effects of the extracts might have influenced the analgesic and local anesthetic actions could not be excluded (Jamieson and Duffield, 1990a).

The local anesthetic activity of topically applied kavain on the rabbit cornea was more pronounced than that of methysticin, with the unhydrated kavalactones kavain and methysticin being more effective than the hydrated analogues, dihydrokavain and dihydromethysticin. While yangonin in a 1% suspension was ineffective, a 0.5% solution of kavain had an effect equivalent to that of 0.5% cocaine. A 3% solution of both kavain and cocaine had a comparable effect on the duration of total anesthesia, extending it from 5.3 to 7.5 minutes to about 31 minutes. The kavalactones in general showed a somewhat weaker infiltration anesthetic effect in comparison to surface anesthetic action. Furthermore, the opioid antagonist naloxone, in doses which inhibited morphine-induced analgesia in both tail immersion and hot plate tests, was completely ineffective in reversing the antinociceptive activities of the kava preparations, indicating that kava produced the analgesia via non-opioid mechanisms (Meyer and May, 1964).

Central nervous and peripheral effects

Muscle paralyzing actions

Meyer (1979) demonstrated that the most characteristic central nervous action of all kavalactones was their ability to produce a mephenesin-like muscular relaxation in all species of laboratory animals. The lactones also proved to be considerably more effective than mephenesin in protecting mice from convulsions and death caused by toxic doses of strychnine. Thus, these compounds were speculated to represent a new group of potent, centrally acting skeletal muscle relaxants, probably the first of natural origin. Larger doses produced ataxia and an ascending paralysis without loss of consciousness, followed by complete recovery. In doses causing muscular relaxation, the lactones did not possess a curare-like action on the neuromuscular function (Meyer, 1966). Death after large oral or ip doses was the result of respiratory failure. In addition, the lactones reduced the edema produced by formalin, serotonin, dextran, and carrageenan. Contractions of isolated ileum or uterus produced by histamine, barium ions, acetylcholine, bradykinin, serotonin, or nicotine were inhibited by the lactones in concentrations $1:10^6-1:10^5$ (Meyer, 1979).

Motor control by mice was assessed either by placing them on a vertical grid and the number of animals unable to remain on the grid was recorded. The animals were also tested on a rotating drum and scored for their ability to retain their equilibrium position on top of the drum which was rotated at 3 rev/min for 1 minute. Aqueous kava extract in dosages up to 250 mg/kg ip had negligible effect on motor control in both tests. However, kava resin (120–250 mg/kg ip) produced a dose-dependent reduction in the ability of the mice to grip and remain on the grid or to remain in the equilibrium position on the rotating drum ($P < 0.005$) (Duffield and Jamieson, 1988; Jamieson *et al.*, 1989). Yangonin (5–10 mg/kg iv) caused an almost total suppression of impulses of the electromyogram. Two- to three-fold higher dosages were required for kavain, methysticin, and dihydromethysticin to produce similar results (Kretzschmar *et al.*, 1971). The muscle relaxing effects of kavalactones have been attributed to a centrally induced attenuation of the α- and γ-spinal motor systems. These effects, similar to those caused by mephenesin, occurred at supraspinal sites of action (Meyer and Kretszchmar, 1966).

The effects of whole kava extract on muscle contractility and neuromuscular transmission were examined by Singh (1983) using *in vitro* twitch tension and electrophysiological techniques. The extent of muscle paralysis was similar in both directly and indirectly stimulated mouse diaphragms. The neuromuscular blockade produced was poorly reversed by calcium and neostigmine. Intracellular recordings showed that kava depressed amplitude of miniature endplate potentials (mepps) and endplate potentials (epps) but had no effect on mepp frequency. Kava also greatly prolonged the duration of mepps and epps. In the isolated frog sartorius muscle, kava was found first to depress the directly elicited muscle action potential and prolong its relaxation phase, then to block the electrical excitability of the membrane (Figure 6.1). These results led the author to conclude that kava caused muscle paralysis by mechanisms similar to local anesthetics like lidocaine. This view is supported by recent observations that various kavalactones effectively block voltage-dependent Na^+ ion channels (Gleitz *et al.*, 1996a,b; Magura *et al.*, 1997).

Spontaneous motility or apomorphine-induced and amphetamine-induced motility in mice were significantly reduced ($P < 0.005$) by aqueous kava extract (62.5–250 mg/kg) and kava resin (120–250 mg/kg). In addition, the two preparations produced a significant reversal ($P < 0.001$) of tetrabenazine-induced ptosis (Duffield *et al.*, 1989a,b). However, the kava effects were smaller compared to those produced by the standard antipsychotic drugs chlorpromazine and haloperidol.

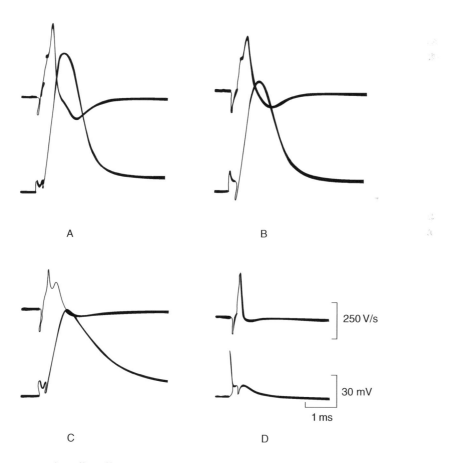

Figure 6.1 Effect of kava (20 mg/ml) on directly evoked muscle action potentials in the isolated frog sartorius muscle preparation before (A), and 20 minutes (B), 40 minutes (C), and 60 minutes (D)
after incubation with the drug. The lower record is the change in transmembrane potential of
the muscle and the upper record is the first derivative of the muscle action potential.
Reprinted from Singh (1983) Effects of kava on neuromuscular transmission and muscle contractility. *Journal of Ethnopharmacology*, 7, 267–276, with permission from Elsevier Science.

Seitz *et al.* (1997b) investigated the effects of (±)-kavain on agonist-evoked contractile activity of isolated guinea-pig ileum. Table 6.1 shows the IC_{50} values of the inhibitory effects of (±)-kavain on muscle contractions evoked by submaximal concentrations (which produce 90–95% of maximal response, E_{max}) of carbachol (10 μM), BAY K 8644 (0.3 μM), or substance P (0.05 μM). The effect of (±)-kavain on contractions evoked by the three agonists was concentration-dependent in the range between 1 μM and 1 mM.

In order to determine if (±)-kavain had calcium channel blocking properties, experiments using nifedipine were performed (Table 6.1). Nifedipine inhibited contractions evoked by BAY K 8644 and by substance P. Even at high concentrations (1 μM), nifedipine failed to completely block contractions evoked by carbachol (10 μM). After pre-incubation with 1 μM nifedipine, carbachol (10 μM) evoked 18.2±4.3% contraction of pre-incubation control value. The remaining response was completely abolished by high concentrations of (±)-kavain (400 μM).

(±)-Kavain also inhibited the contractile responses induced by raising the extracellular K^+ concentration from 4 to 20 mM or by blocking the K^+ channels with barium chloride (1 mM) or 4-aminopyridine (0.3 μM). The IC_{50} values for (±)-kavain on depolarization-induced contractions by potassium (20 mM), barium chloride (1 mM), and 4-aminopyridine (0.3 μM) were 52.5 μM, 30.8 μM, and 44.3 μM, respectively. After treatment of the longitudinal ileum strips with pertussis toxin, carbachol (1 μM) evoked 27.0±6.2% of the control response in untreated ileum. These contractions were also blocked by (±)-kavain (400 μM). However, (±)-kavain had no effect on caffeine-induced (20 mM) contractions in ileum strips which had been permeabilized with digitonin or β-escin. Moreover, it failed to affect Ca^{2+}-evoked contractions of skinned muscles. These results suggest that (±)-kavain acts directly on the smooth muscle membrane in a non-specific musculotropic manner.

Visual effects

In a study on the visual effects produced by kava, Garner and Klinger (1985) noted a reduced near point of accommodation and convergence, an increase in pupil diameter and a disturbance to the oculomotor balance. However, no changes were recorded in

Table 6.1 Comparison of the inhibition of experimentally induced contractions of the isolated guinea pig ileum by (±)-kavain and nifedipine

Agonist *(Submaximal concentration)*	*(±)-Kavain* *(IC_{50})*	*Nifedipine* *(IC_{50})*
Carbachol (10 μM)	144.0 μM	n.d.
Bay K 8644 (0.3 μM)	29.3 μM	5.7 nM
Substance P (0.05 μM)	54.7 μM	6.7 nM

Sources: Seitz *et al.* (1997) Relaxation of evoked contractile activity of isolated guinea pig ileum by (±)-kavain. *Planta Medica*, **63**, 303–306, with permission from Georg Thieme Verlag.

Notes
The IC_{50} values are the concentrations that reduced the agonist-induced concentration of the ileum by 50%. Agonists were employed at submaximal concentrations, i.e., 90–95% of maximal contractions, E_{max}.
n.d. – not determined.

visual or stereoacuity, or in ocular refractive error. The exact mechanism of the changes in accommodation could be due to a direct muscle action or a vascular response, which would be consistent with a local anesthetic type action as previously proposed (Singh, 1983). Alternatively, the visual and ocular effects of kava may also be under central nervous control, and therefore show some variation under the control of this beverage. The near point of convergence and accommodation requires considerable voluntary effort and it could be that a central sedative effect was being measured for these functions. In the case of the pupil size, the increase in diameter may be due to a direct muscle action, as suggested above, or may reflect a central activity of kava. However, the disturbance to oculomotor balance could only be explained in terms of central nervous changes (Garner and Klinger, 1985).

Information processing and cognition

In a placebo-controlled study, the effects of kava on alertness and speed of accessing of information in long-term memory was evaluated in two groups of naïve drinkers who consumed doses thought usual or greater than those used at social functions in the South Pacific. Neither the imbibing of 250 mL of the kava beverage, prepared from 30 g of pulverized rhizome, nor the ingestion of a double dose, led to impairment of reaction, memory, or motor coordination (Russell *et al.*, 1987). Using a battery of cognitive and visuomotor tests, Foo and Lemon (1997) also could not detect any kava-induced impairment in performance skills in a group of 40 subjects. In a randomized single blind 14 day study, six healthy volunteers were given either 300 or 600 mg daily of kava extract, which were equivalent to daily doses of 210 and 420 mg kavalactones, respectively.

The efficacy of kava was further gauged by examining the neurophysiological spectrum of actions comprised of quantitative EEG and evoked potentials, general personality variables and the subjective state, including a variety of cognitive parameters. An increase in the beta/alpha-index in the quantitative EEG was present, which is typical for the pharmaco-EEG profile of anxiolytics (Buchsbaum *et al.*, 1985). Delta and theta activity were unchanged, signifying the absence of a sedative component. The data pertaining to the evoked potentials indicated an improvement in attentiveness and information processing in the cortical areas. The analysis of the various parameters also indicated an increased tendency towards emotional stability (Johnson *et al.*, 1991).

Saletu *et al.* (1989) used a double-blind, placebo-controlled study to evaluate the encephalotropic and psychotropic effects of synthetic kavain and the benzodiazepine clobazam, utilizing EEG brain mapping and psychometric analysis. Brain maps of drug-induced pharmaco-EEG changes demonstrated that kavain exerted a significant action on the human brain function characterized by a dose-dependent increase in delta, theta and alpha 1 activity. These findings are indicative of a sedative effect. Psychometric data indicated that kavain produced significant improvement compared to placebo ($P < 0.05$) in intellectual performance (Pauli test), attention, mental concentration, reaction time, and motor speed, while the opposite findings were obtained with clobazam.

Prescott *et al.* (1993) investigated the acute effects of kava on 24 volunteers (11 males and 13 females, mean age 26.7 years, range 18–53 years) who either consumed a kava beverage or a placebo drink. The kava liquid provided the equivalent of 100 g per person of powdered Fijian kava root prepared in a manner which approximated the traditional infusion techniques. A comparison of the kava and placebo groups revealed a low-to-moderate degree of intoxication, which peaked in about one hour. There was a statistically significant increase ($P < 0.05$) in body sway, but no effect on respiration rate, heart rate, blood pressure, or stress levels. However, the group receiving kava had an insignificant tendency to impaired performance on more complex tests of cognitive function. Chemical analysis showed that the kava group consumed an average of 228 mg of dihydrokavain (range 129–317 g) and 225 g of kavain (range 129–317 g).

The influence of kava extract, alone or in combination with alcohol or bromazepam, on safety-related performance has been investigated in some human pharmacological studies. In a placebo-controlled, randomized, double-blind, eight day study (Herberg, 1993), 20 healthy subjects daily received three divided doses of 100 mg kava extract (WS 1490), which was equivalent to a total of 210 mg kavalactones, or a placebo. Seven psychometric testing procedures were implemented in investigating the safety-related performance. There were no statistically significant differences ($P > 0.05$) detected when comparing the kava group to the placebo group with regard to vigilance, optic orientation, mental concentration, reaction time, or motor coordination. When ethanol (blood alcohol concentration or BAC of 0.05%) was co-administered with the kava extract on days 1, 4, and 8 of the test, there was no synergistic effect with the combination. In a subsequent randomized, double-blind, crossover study, 18 healthy persons were given individually or in combination, 400 mg kava extract (equivalent to 240 mg kavalactones daily) and 4.5 mg bromazepam twice daily for eight days (Herberg, 1996). For the performance parameters, there were some extremely significant differences ($P < 0.001$). Performance in stress tolerance, vigilance, and motor coordination with kava extract remained at the baseline level, while they deteriorated considerably in the subjects taking bromazepam or the kava-bromazepam combination. The data for bromazepam and the combination did not differ from one another. The least impairment of wellbeing was seen in the treatment with kava extract, while the greatest impairment of wellbeing was present in the combination treatment. There were no clear indications of synergistic interactions when the substances were given in combination.

In a placebo-controlled, randomized, double-blind, three-fold crossover clinical study, 12 healthy volunteers were evaluated for the effects of a single dose of kava extract equivalent to 120 mg kavalactones and 10 mg diazepam. Measurements were taken directly before, and two and six hours post ingestion. The washout period before crossover was seven days. After kava administration, a non-significant increase compared to placebo was noted in the quantitative EEG in the delta/theta intensity in the occipital and frontal areas, as well as a reduction of the alpha-wave relative intensity ($P < 0.05$). An increase in beta activity typically found with benzodiazepines was not observed with kava. The placebo group witnessed a decline in the relative intensity of the slow delta- and theta-waves and an increase in the alpha-waves ($P < 0.001$). Maximal effects of diazepam were usually observed two hours after application, as opposed to the kava extract where the effects had not decreased even after six hours. The critical flicker frequency in the psychophysiological tests was found to be lower under the influence of kava extract and diazepam compared to placebo ($P < 0.05$). In contrast, significant increases in performance in the Pauli Test after the administration of kava extract were noted which were not present with the placebo or diazepam ($P < 0.05$) (Gessner and Cnota, 1994).

Twelve healthy volunteers were tested in a placebo-controlled double-blind crossover study to assess the effects of oxazepam and a standardized extract of kava rhizome (WS1490) on behavior and event-related potentials (ERPs) in a word recognition task.

The test group received 600 mg kava extract daily in three divided doses (equivalent to 420 mg kavalactones daily) over the course of five days; the placebo group received three doses daily; while the oxazepam group received the placebo from day 1 to 4 followed by 15 mg oxazepam on the evening of day 4 and 75 mg oxazepam on day 5. The duration of study was 29 days, and between the three 5-day therapy sessions there were wash-out periods of seven days. The word recognition task (employed as a parameter for memory performance) and psychometric tests were used to examine ERPs. Oxazepam produced a statistically significant attenuation in cerebral information processing and an amplitude increase with corresponding changes in the ERPs, the repeated recognition rate, and psychometric tests ($P < 0.05$). In contrast, the kava extract resulted in a slight but non-significant increase in the word recognition rate and amplitude of the ERPs ($P > 0.05$) (Münte *et al.*, 1993).

The effects of oxazepam and a standardized extract of kava roots (WS1490) on reaction time and ERPs were investigated in a visual search paradigm using a double-blind randomized crossover design in 20 young, healthy male subjects. In a five day study period, the subjects were given three divided doses of 200 mg/kg of kava or placebo for five days, or pretreated with 15 mg of oxazepam the evening before and then 75 mg on the morning of the test day. The experimental sessions were 12 days apart to allow ample washout time for the drugs. Several ERP components of different latency, topography, and functional significance were affected by the medications. Oxazepam led to a reduction in the amplitude of the parietal N1, frontal N2, posterior contralateral N2, and occipital P3 components, suggesting deficits in automatic feature registration, allocation of attention, and the available processing capacity. Kava was, on the other hand, associated with a greater posterior N1, posterior contralateral N2, and occipital P3, indicating a positive effect on the allocation of attention and processing capacity (Heinze *et al.*, 1994).

The lack of a negative effect by kava and its constituents on information processing and cognition is consistent with various historic ethnographic accounts of kava use in earlier times. For instance, Morrison, who visited Tahiti between 1788 and 1791, wrote, "(Kava)...deprives them of the use of their limbs and speech, but does not touch the mental faculty and they appear in a thoughtful mood and frequently fall backwards before they have finished eating. Some of their attendants then attend to chafe their limbs all over until they fall asleep. After a few hours they are as fresh as if nothing had happened and are ready for another dose" (Morrison, 1935). Hocart (1929) noted that "it gives a pleasant, warm and cheerful, but lazy feeling, sociable, though not hilarious or loquacious; the reason is not obscured." According to Lemert (1967) "The head is affected pleasantly; you feel friendly, not beer sentimental; you cannot hate with kava in you. Kava quiets the mind; the world gains no rosy tint; it fits in its place and in one easily understandable whole."

Because of the preceding evidence for the effects of kava on cognitive functions and information processing, and as long-term potentiation (LTP) is a widely accepted model for learning, memory, and synaptic plasticity (Bliss and Collingridge, 1993), an investigation was done to clarify whether the mechanism of action of kava is in part dependent on an effect on LTP. Hence the effects of (±)-kavain on LTP were tested in the CA1 region of guinea pig hippocampal slices (Langosch *et al.*, 1998). As Figure 6.2 shows, (±)-kavain (1–300 µM) reversibly reduced the amplitudes of extracellular field potential changes evoked by electrical stimulation in a concentration dependent manner. However, in experiments with LTP, no changes were observed in the presence

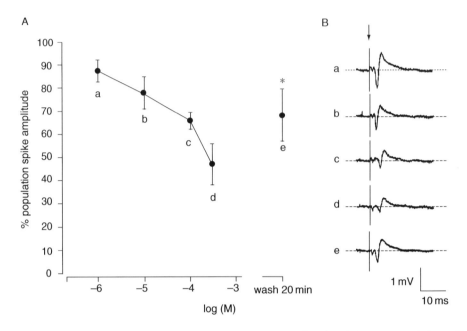

Figure 6.2 Decrease of field potential changes (population spikes) by (±)-kavain. Population spikes were evoked by constant current stimulation of the Schaffer collateral pathway and detected in the striatum pyramidale of the CA1 region of hippocampus. (A) The concentration–response curve was obtained by applying increasing concentrations of the drug for 10 minutes (1–300 μM). The interval between subsequent applications was 15 minutes. Washout values were measured 20 minutes after finishing (±)-kavain applications. Means ± S.E.M. from six experiments. *$P < 0.05$, significant difference between d and e. Representative tracings from one experiment are shown in (B). Arrow indicates stimuli. Reprinted from Langosch *et al.* (1998) The influence of (±)-kavain on population spikes and long-term potentiation in guinea pig hippocampal slices. *Comparative Biochemistry and Physiology*, **120**, 545–549, with permission from Elsevier Science.

of the lactone. The findings indicate that (±)-kavain is effective in modulating excitatory signals in the hippocampus, but no alterations in synaptic plasticity can be assumed for the compound.

Anticonvulsant actions

Many studies have shown that kava extract and the kavalactones present in it have anti-convulsant effects in mice with experimentally induced tonic-extensor convulsions, produced by maximal electroshock, strychnine, pentylenetetrazol, bemegride, and picrotoxin (Klohs *et al.*, 1959; Meyer, 1964; Kretzschmar *et al.*, 1969; Kretzschmar and Meyer, 1969) Methysticin and dihydromethysticin proved to be the most effective in this respect. As kavalactones are poorly absorbed in the gut, the oral administration of unsaturated kavalactones required a dosage that was ten-fold higher than that required by intravenous administration. Mixtures of yangonin or desmethoxyyangonin with 5,6-hydrated lactones (kavain, dihydrokavain, methysticin, and dihydromethysticin) administered po led to a synergistic effect. The mean protective dosage against the maximal electroshock was 740 mg/kg po for yangonin. However, this amount decreased to 75 mg/kg when yangonin was administered in a 1:1 ratio with the kavalactone mixture consisting of kavain, dihydrokavain, methysticin, and dihydromethysticin in equal proportions. This dosage for yangonin was much less than the calculated estimate of 115.2 mg/kg (Kretzschmar and Teschendorf, 1974), indicating the presence of a synergistic effect. After po administration, kavain activity peaked at 10 minutes and the activity lasted for 40–60 minutes. Methysticin activity peaked at 45–60 minutes with an activity period of 2–4 hours, while yangonin activity peaked at 2 hours (Kretzschmar and Meyer, 1969).

The effects of methysticin on three different *in vitro* models of seizure-like events were studied in rat hippocampal and entorhinal slices. Methysticin, in concentrations ranging from 10 to 100 μM, blocked all types of epileptiform discharges induced in all experiments. This included stimulus induced burst discharges in low Mg^{2+}, all types of low Mg^{2+} induced recurrent activities in the entorhinal cortex, and the low Ca^{2+}, as well as the high K^+ induced epileptiform discharges in area CA1 of the hippocampus. The findings suggest that methysticin has effects on different patterns of epileptiform activity possibly by interfering with processes responsible for frequency potentiation (Schmitz *et al.*, 1995).

Additionally, the kava resin and purified dihydromethysticin, when tested for anticonvulsant activity in humans, provided some control of grand mal seizures in one trial (Pfeiffer *et al.*, 1979). However, other workers (Jamieson *et al.*, 1989) found that the anticonvulsant effect of the aqueous extract against strychnine was very slight. From this and other observations it appears that many of the pharmacological effects of kava appear to be mainly due to the activity of the compounds present in the lipid soluble resin fraction.

Neuroprotection

Cerebral ischemia and neuronal damage can be caused by excessive release of excitatory amino acids (Benveniste *et al.*, 1984), and blockers of neuronal stimulation, such as anticonvulsants, are capable of protecting brain tissue against ischemic damage (Meldrum *et al.*, 1985). In light of these observations and the anticonvulsant action of kavalactones, Backhauss and Krieglstein (1992a,b) investigated whether kava extract and its constituents could provide protection against ischemic brain damage. Memantine was included in the study as a typical anticonvulsant. Kava extract (150 mg po, containing 70% kavalactones) administered to mice 1 hour before the occlusion of the middle cerebral artery reduced the cerebral infarct size ($P < 0.05$) in mouse brains and the infarct volume ($P < 0.05$) in rat brains. Methysticin (10 mg/kg ip) and dihydromethysticin (30 mg/kg ip) 15 minutes before ischemia, and memantine (20 mg/kg ip) 30 minutes before ischemia, displayed approximately the same significant neuroprotective effects, whereas kavain, dihydrokavain, and yangonin had no influence. These workers also examined the effects of kava extract and its various constituents on primary neuronal cell cultures prepared from seven-day old chick embryo cerebral hemispheres and tested under cytotoxic hypoxia conditions. As in the *in vivo* experiments, only the kava extract, methysticin, and dihydromethysticin provided protection, prompting the authors to conclude that the neuroprotective effect of the extract was mediated by methysticin and dihydromethysticin in the kava extract acting directly on neurons (Backhauss and Krieglstein, 1992b).

There are reports that blockers of voltage-dependent Na^+ channels, such as local anesthetics, can reduce infarct size (Rataud *et al.*, 1994) and diminish the neuronal damage following reduction in cerebral blood flow (Yamasaki *et al.*, 1991). Because the kavalactones are known to block Na^+ channels, the influence of (±)-kavain and the Na^+ channel blocker tetrodotoxin on anoxic rat brain vesicles was examined with respect to lactate synthesis, vesicular ATP content, and cytosolic free Na^+ and Ca^{2+} ([Na^+]i, [Ca^{2+}]i). (±)-Kavain or tetrodotoxin, if applied before anoxia, preserved vesicular ATP content, diminished anoxia-induced increase in [Na^+]i and [Ca^{2+}]i and prevented both the veratridine-induced increases of [Na^+]i and [Ca^{2+}]i and the inhibition of lactate production, thus counteracting the adverse effects which would otherwise occur in damaged neurons (Gleitz *et al.*, 1996c).

Studies on other effects

The antimicrobial properties of the kavalactones have been studied (Hänsel, 1968). A large number of Gram-positive, Gram-negative, pathogenic, and non-pathogenic bacteria were found to grow uninhibited in nutrients containing the lactones, indicating they were not bacteriostatic in nature. On the other hand, some of the lactones showed remarkable fungistatic properties against a wide genera of fungi, including some which were pathogenic to humans. These findings were recently confirmed by Locher *et al.* (1995) who, in addition, found no anti-viral activity with kava extract when tested against Herpes Simplex-1 and -2, Semliki Forest, Vesicular Stomatitis, Polio, and Coxsackie B3 viruses.

The assumed antithrombotic action of (±)-kavain on human platelets was deduced from its ability to suppress arachidonic acid (AA)-induced platelet aggregation, exocytosis of ATP, and inhibition of cyclooxygenase-2 (COX-2) and thromboxane synthase (TXS) activity, the latter two effects being estimated from the generation of prostaglandin E_2 (PGE_2) and thromboxane A_2 (TXA_2), respectively. Exogenously-applied AA (100 μM) provoked a 90% aggregation of platelets, the release of 14 pmol ATP, and the formation of either 43 pg PGE_2 or 220 pg TXA_2, each parameter being related to 10^6 platelets. (±)-Kavain dose-dependently suppressed the aggregation of human platelets (IC_{50} 78 μM), the release of endogenous ATP (IC_{50} 115 μM), and the formation of prostaglandin E_2 (IC_{50} 86 μM) and thromboxane A_2 (IC_{50} 71 μM). The similarity of the IC_{50} values suggests an inhibition of COX-2 by (±)-kavain as a primary target, thus suppressing the exocytosis of ATP by its binding on the COX-2 receptors and generation of TXA_2 which induces aggregation of platelets (Gleitz *et al.*, 1997).

To clarify the mechanism by which kava exerts its reputed psychotropic properties, the *in vitro* effects of a kava extract and pure synthetic kavalactones were investigated on human platelet monoamine oxidase-B (MAO-B), in comparison to amitriptyline, imipramine, and brofaromine (Uebelhack *et al.*, 1998). The kava extract (67.6% kavalactones) was added to assay mixtures, containing platelet-rich plasma (PRP), to achieve final concentrations in the range of 2–225 μM for intact platelets in PRP or 0.25–0.45 μM for disrupted platelets. Synthetic kavalactones were tested at a concentration of 20 μM for intact platelets. The final concentration of (±)-kavain, desmethoxyyangonin, and (±)-methysticin were varied in the range 0.05–200 μM to determine the IC_{50} values. For kinetic studies, disrupted platelets were incubated with either (±)-methysticin or desmethoxyyangonin (1–16 μM). Table 6.2 shows the IC_{50} values of two antidepressants,

Table 6.2 Inhibition of PEA deamination in platelets by kava–kava extract, some kavalactones, antidepressants and brofaromine ($n=4$)

	IC_{50} (μM) Intact platelets	IC_{50} (μM) Disrupted platelets
($\pm$)-kavain	>400	40.5 ± 10.6
($\pm$)-methysticin	39.5 ± 17.9	0.67 ± 0.12
desmethoxyyangonin	28.1 ± 12.9	0.12 ± 0.02
kava–kava extract	24.0 ± 12.4	1.4 ± 0.6
amitriptyline	33.2 ± 12.8	12.7 ± 6.6
imipramine	41.2 ± 10.6	21.7 ± 10.8
brofaromine	23.7 ± 6.5	10.0 ± 5.3

Source: Uebelhack *et al.* (1998). Inhibition of platelet MAO-B by kava-pyrone-enriched extract from *Piper methysticum* Forster (kava–kava). *Pharmacopsychiatry*, 31, 187–192, with permission from Georg Thieme Verlag.

Notes
PEA – 2-phenylethylamine-[ethyl-1-^{14}C]hydrochloride.

brofaromine, kava extract and kavalactones for the inhibition of 2-phenylethylamine-[ethyl-1-^{14}C]hydrochloride (PEA) deamination in intact and disrupted platelets.

All substances appeared to be about equipotent in intact platelets, except for ($\pm$)-kavain. A much higher concentration (17–234 times) of kavalactones was required to inhibit MAO-B activity in intact platelets than in disrupted platelets, whereas the antidepressants and brofaromine were only about twice as active in the disrupted platelets. The IC_{50} value of the kava extract in disrupted platelets was about ten times lower than that of either amitriptyline or brofaromine and 20 times lower than that of imipramine. The sensitivity of MAO-B activity to synthetic kavain was very much lower in both preparations. Structural differences of the kavalactones resulted in MAO-B inhibition in the order of potency of desmethoxyyangonin > ($\pm$)-methysticin > yangonin > ($\pm$)-dihydromethysticin > ($\pm$)-dihydrokavain > ($\pm$)-kavain. The two most potent kavalactones, desmethoxyyangonin (IC_{50} 28.1 μM in intact platelets) and ($\pm$)-methysticin (IC_{50} 39.5 μM in intact platelets) displayed a competitive inhibition pattern with mean K_i values of 0.28 μM and 1.14 μM, respectively. As indicated by the IC_{50} value of 40.5 μM, ($\pm$)-kavain was a weak inhibitor of MAO-B in disrupted platelets, while in intact platelets it was not possible to measure its IC_{50} (Uebelhack *et al.*, 1998).

The acute effects of a kava preparation and diazepam were recently examined in an animal model with Wistar rats using the elevated plus X-maze test (Rex *et al.*, 2002). Presently this is the most popular and widely used animal test for anxiety and, in addition, the results obtained can be compared with the literature and rated more easily than previous tests (Hogg, 1996). Kava (LI 150®, Lichtwer, Berlin) in oral dosages of 120 and 180 mg/kg induced an "anxiolytic-like" behavior similar to diazepam (1.5 mg/kg po) and was, like the benzodiazepine, significantly greater than the controls.

Pharmacological Mechanisms of Action

Effects on ion channels

Extensive work has recently been done on the effects of ($\pm$)-kavain on voltage-activated ion channels in synaptosomes prepared from rat cerebral cortex, anoxic rat brain slices, and dorsal root ganglion cells from neonatal rats. The influence of (±)-kavain on veratridine-stimulated increase in Na⁺ concentration ([Na⁺]i) in rat cerebrocortical synaptosomes was studied spectrofluorometrically employing sodium-binding benzo-furanisophthalate (SBFI) as a Na⁺ sensitive fluorescence dye. (±)-Kavain reduced dose-dependently the ouabain-stimulated (200 μM) increase of [Na⁺]i with an IC_{50} value of 86.0 μM, and almost complete inhibition of Na⁺-channels was attained with 400 μM (±)-kavain and the potent Na⁺ channel blocker tetrodotoxin (10 μM) (Figure 6.3). The local anesthetic procaine (400 μM) reduced veratridine-elevated [Na⁺]i to 30.4% of control, whereas the centrally acting muscle relaxant mephenesin (400 μM) produced no effect. The data indicated a fast and specific inhibition of voltage-dependent Na⁺-channels by (±)-kavain (Gleitz *et al.*, 1995).

The interaction of (±)-kavain with receptor site 1 of Na⁺ channels, which is the epitope of antagonists like saxitoxin and tetrodotoxin, and its influence on site 2, the binding site of agonists including veratridine, batrachotoxin, and aconitine, were investigated on cerebrocortical synaptosomes by radioligand-binding assays. 4-Aminopyridine, a K⁺ channel blocker, reduced the membrane potential sufficiently

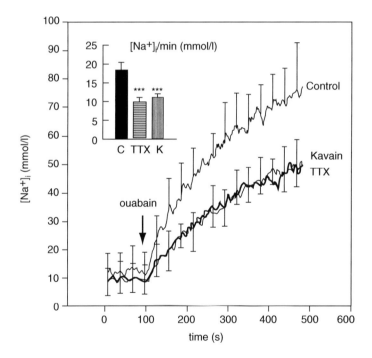

Figure 6.3 Reduction by tetrodotoxin (TTX, 10 μmol/l) and (±)-kavain (400 μmol/l) of ouabain-induced (200 μmol/l) Na⁺ influx into rat cerebrocortical synaptosomes. From top to bottom: Control, (±)-kavain-treated (lower thick-line trace), and TTX-treated (lower thin-line trace). Inset: Increase in [Na⁺]i/min of control (C), TTX and (±)-kavain (K). Traces represent mean ± S.E., *n* = 6, *P* < 0.001. Reprinted from Gleitz *et al.* (1995) (±)-Kavain inhibits the veratridine-activated voltage-dependent Na⁺ channels in synaptosomes prepared from rat cerebral cortex. *Neuropharmacology*, 34, 1133–1138, 1995, with permission from Elsevier Science.

to activate voltage-dependent Na^+ channels, an effect correlated with an increase in cytosolic free $[Na^+]i$ and $[Ca^{2+}]i$, and the release of endogenous glutamate. Glutamate released from the 4-aminopyridine-stimulated synaptosomes and the cytosolic free $[Na^+]i$ and $[Ca^{2+}]i$ were detected fluorometrically by using an enzyme-linked assay, the sodium sensitive dye SBFI, and Fura-2, respectively. ($\pm$)-Kavain failed to compete with $[^3H]$saxitoxin in concentrations up to $400\,\mu M$, but dose-dependently suppressed binding of $[^3H]$batrachotoxin with an IC_{50} value of $88\,\mu M$, although displacement of $[^3H]$batrachotoxin was restricted to 33% of control at $400\,\mu M$ ($\pm$)-kavain (Gleitz *et al.*, 1996b). $100\,\mu M$ ($\pm$)-kavain, $50\,\mu M$ (+)-kavain, $70\,\mu M$ ($\pm$)-dihydrokavain, $100\,\mu M$ (+)-dihydrokavain, and $100\,\mu M$ (+)-dihydromethysticin decreased ($P < 0.01$) the apparent total number of binding sites (B_{max}) for $[^3H]$batrachotoxinin-A, while the K_D value for each compound was not significantly affected (Friese and Gleitz, 1998). In synaptosomes stimulated by 4-aminopyridine ($5\,\mu M$), ($\pm$)-kavain ($400\,\mu M$) suppressed the increases in $[Na^+]i$ and $[Ca^{2+}]i$ to 38 and 29% of control, respectively. In KCl-depolarized synaptosomes, ($\pm$)-kavain ($400\,\mu M$) reduced KCl-evoked $[Ca^{2+}]i$ elevation and diminished the part of glutamate exocytosis which is related to external Ca^{2+} to about 75% of control (Gleitz *et al.*, 1996b).

In a related study, Gleitz *et al.* (1996d) examined the actions of the natural kavalactone, ($\pm$)-kavain, and its synthetic racemate, ($\pm$)-kavain, on veratridine-induced increases in $[Na^+]i$ and $[Ca^{2+}]i$ and the release of endogenous glutamate from cerebrocortical synaptosomes. As shown in Figure 6.4 inserts, the two kavains had very little effect on basal levels of $[Na^+]i$, and $[Ca^{2+}]i$ or spontaneous glutamate release. Stimulation of the synaptosomes with veratridine provoked an appreciable increase in the cation levels, which leveled off 200–300 s after veratridine application, and in glutamate release. However, pretreatment of the preparations with the kavains 100 s before veratridine application dose-dependently suppressed the increases in $[Na^+]i$ and $[Ca^{2+}]i$. It was found that both kavalactones suppressed increases in the cation levels (Figure 6.4) with similar IC_{50} values, while IC_{50} values with respect to glutamate release were not significantly different ($P > 0.05$) (Table 6.3), indicating a non-stereospecific inhibition of Na^+ ion channels. Indirect evidence for a non-stereospecific inhibition of Na^+ ion channels was previously provided by Meyer and Kretzschmar (1969) who demonstrated equal efficacy for intravenously administered ($\pm$)-kavain and (+)-kavain against electroshock-induced convulsions.

These effects of ($\pm$)-kavain on voltage-activated Na^+ and Ca^{2+} inward currents were analyzed by patch clamp technique in cultured dorsal root ganglion cells from neonatal

Table 6.3 IC_{50} values of (+)-kavain and ($\pm$)-kavain for the inhibition of veratridine-induced increases in $[Na^+]_i$, $[Ca^{2+}]_i$, and glutamate release. Data are means $\pm$ S.D. ($n = 6$)

Parameter	IC_{50} (μmol/l) (+)-*Kavain*	IC_{50} (μmol/l) ($\pm$)-*Kavain*
$\Delta[Na^+]_i$	71 ± 22	77 ± 21
$\Delta[Ca^{2+}]_i$	77 ± 7	90 ± 14
Glutamate release	120 ± 37	92 ± 23

Source: Gleitz *et al.* (1996a) Kavain inhibits non-stereospecifically veratridine activated Na^+ channels. *Planta Medica*, **62**, 580–581, with permission from Georg Thieme Verlag.

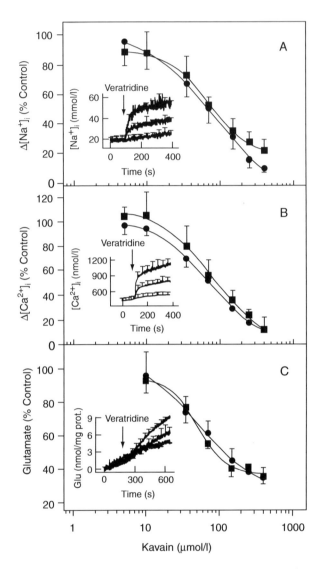

Figure 6.4 Inhibition of veratridine-induced increases in $[Na^+]_i$, $[Ca^{2+}]_i$, and glutamate release by kavain. In the example shown for (+)-kavain in the insets, the addition of (±)-kavain (■) or (+)-kavain (●) 100s before veratridine (5 μmol/l) dose-dependently suppressed the increase in $[Na^+]_i$ (A), $[Ca^{2+}]_i$ (B) and the release of glutamate (C). Traces from top to bottom represent means ± S.D. ($n = 6$) of (1) control, (2) 70 μmol/l (+)-kavain, and (3) 400 μmol/l (+)-kavain. Data are depicted as means ± S.D. ($n = 6$). Reprinted from Gleitz *et al.* (1996a) Kavain inhibits non-stereospecifically veratridine-activated Na^+ channels. *Planta Medica*, 62, 580–581, with permission from Elsevier Science.

rats using the whole cell configuration. Extracellularly applied (±)-kavain reduced currents through voltage-activated Na^+ and Ca^{2+} channels within 3–5 minutes (Schirrmacher *et al.*, 1999). A comparative study of the actions of the natural kavalactone, (+)-kavain, and its synthetic racemate, (±)-kavain, on veratridine-induced increases in

$[Na^+]i$ and $[Ca^{2+}]i$ and the release of endogenous glutamate from cerebrocortical synaptosomes found that both kavalactones were equally effective, confirming a non-stereospecific inhibition of veratridine-activated Na^+ channels (Gleitz *et al.*, 1996a).

Recently, Martin and coworkers have shown that (±)-kavain attenuates rodent smooth muscle contraction. In isolated isometrically contracted murine tracheal preparations, kavain diminished the contractile responses to both muscarinic receptor stimulation as well as voltage-gated calcium channel activation (Martin *et al.*, 2000). The IC_{50} for kavain in rings precontracted with carbachol was found to be $177 \pm 53.1\,\mu M$, and, in rings precontracted with KCl, it was $59.6 \pm 10.1\,\mu M$. In addition, pretreatment with kavain attenuated the muscle contraction evoked both with carbachol or KCl. The EC_{50} for KCl was not affected by kava pretreatment. However, the IC_{50} for carbachol was significantly increased by a high kava pretreatment dose. Nitric oxide mediated relaxation was not observed to play a role in kavain's smooth muscle relaxing properties. Similarly, prostaglandin pathways are unlikely to be involved in these effects since pretreatment of tracheal rings with indomethacin before carbachol contraction did not affect the relaxant effect of kavain. The authors concluded that the mechanism of kavain-induced relaxation was likely due to a mechanism common to both contractile agonists used in the study, namely carbachol and KCl.

Martin *et al.* (2002) also found that (±)-kavain (10^{-6}–$10^{-3}\,M$) dose-dependently relaxed isolated rat aortic ring preparations that had previously been contracted with phenylephrine (PE), as an effect not dependent on functional epithelium. In addition, kavain pretreatment attenuated muscle contraction evoked by PE. However, PE elicited contraction in Ca^{2+} free buffer was not affected by kavain, suggesting that intracellular signaling mechanisms probably were not involved. In rings pretreated with the L-type Ca^{2+} channel blocker nifedipine, kavain mediated relaxation was appreciably attenuated. Further, muscles selectively contracted with Bay K 8644, an L-type Ca^{2+} channel activator, were dose-dependently relaxed by kavain. The findings suggest that kavain impairs vascular smooth muscle contraction probably through inhibition of Ca^{2+} ion channels.

A microdialysis study in freely moving rats confirmed the earlier *in vivo* effects of (±)-kavain on veratridine-induced glutamate release (Ferger *et al.*, 1998). (±)-Kavain (100 mg/kg po) significantly reduced veratridine-induced glutamate release compared to that in vehicle-treated control animals. Maximum extracellular glutamate levels were obtained 20–40 minutes after stimulation with veratridine ($500\,\mu M$) added to the perfusate. In the control group the increase was 301% of basal extracellular glutamate level, while in the (±)-kavain group the increase was significantly reduced to 219% ($P < 0.01$). The coperfusion of veratridine ($500\,\mu M$) and tetrodotoxin ($5\,\mu M$) led to an almost complete suppression of veratridine-induced glutamate release after 40 minutes and served as a positive control.

The action of (+)-methysticin and (±)-kavain on voltage-generated Na^+ channels was studied in whole-cell patch-clamped CA1 hippocampal neurons. In doses of 1–400 μM, both compounds exerted a rapid and reversible inhibition of the peak amplitude of Na^+ currents. Shifting of the holding membrane potential (V_{hold}) to more positive values enhanced their blocking effects. The two compounds did not demonstrate use-dependent properties at 10 Hz stimulation but shifted h_∞ curve toward more negative potentials, accelerated time-course of inactivation, and slowed down the recovery from inactivation. Furthermore, compared to (±)-kavain, (+)-methysticin was about a four- to five-fold more potent blocker of peak current amplitude at different V_{hold} values and caused a larger shift of h_∞ curve towards more negative potentials. The authors concluded that the considerable voltage-dependence of Na^+ channel inhibition by (+)-methysticin and (±)-kavain was due to their interaction with resting closed and inactivated states of the Na^+ channel (Magura *et al.*, 1997).

Effects on GABA and benzodiazepine receptors

In order to elucidate the anxiolytic and sedating properties of kava, Jamieson's group studied the interaction of kava resin and $100\,\mu M$ and $1\,mM$ of the purified kavalactones kavain, dihydrokavain, methysticin, dihydromethysticin, yangonin, and tetrahydro-yangonin, with GABA and benzodiazepine receptor binding sites in rat and mouse brain membranes. No binding was observed at $GABA_B$ receptors and there was only weak activity at $GABA_A$ receptors in washed synaptosomal membranes from rat forebrain and cerebellum (Davies *et al.*, 1992). The weak binding at $GABA_A$ receptors was abolished by extraction of the membranes with Triton-X, suggesting that only lipid soluble components were involved. The kava resin and the kava lactones exerted some weak effects on benzodiazepine binding *in vitro* but this did not correlate with pharmacological activity. In *ex vivo* studies, no effects were observed on $[^3H]$diazepam binding to brain membranes prepared from mice in which selected kava constituents had been injected ip, whereas similarly administered diazepam (5 mg/kg) inhibited $[^3H]$ diazepam binding by >95%. Furthermore, injection of kava resin failed to influence the CNS binding of the benzodiazepine receptor ligand $[^3H]$Ro15–1788 injected into mice prior to sacrifice. The authors concluded that the pharmacological activities of the kava preparations were not due to direct interactions of the kavalactones with the benzodiazepine or $GABA_A$ receptor, rather that the lipophilic kavalactones were incorporated into the lipid membranes, leading to a non-specific modification of the $GABA_A$ receptor conformation (Davies *et al.*, 1992).

In contrast, Boonen and Haberlein (1998) found there was substantial binding of genuine kavalactones enantiomers on the $GABA_A$ receptor site. Radioreceptor assays were performed using freeze-dried rat cortex preparations bearing the $GABA_A$ receptor, and the radioligand $[^3H]$bicuculline methochloride ($[^3H]$BMC). The radioreceptor assay was verified by an in-process procedure with an increase of specific $[^3H]$BMC binding of about 14% using diazepam (10 nM) and an IC_{50} value for bicuculline methoiodide of 50 nM. (+)-Kavain, (+)-methysticin, and (+)-dihydromethysticin showed maximal enhancements of the specific $[^3H]$BMC binding of 18–28 % at a concentration of $0.1\,\mu M$, whereas a 100-fold higher concentration of (+)-dihydrokavain was needed for a similar modulatory activity of 22% ($P < 0.01$). In the presence of $1\,\mu M$ yangonin, an increase of about 21% ($P < 0.01$) of specific $[^3H]$BMC binding was observed, but desmethoxyyangonin did not alter the binding behavior of the $GABA_A$ receptor.

It is evident that the aromatic methoxy group in kavalactones is of particular importance for the modulatory activity of the dienolides. From a comparison of the molecular structures of (+)-kavain and desmethoxyyangonin, it is evident that an angular lactone ring lacking a double bond is a crucial structural requirement for the enolides in order for them to alter the binding behavior of the $GABA_A$ receptor. The modulatory activity of the kavalactones at assay concentrations between $0.1\,\mu M$ and $10\,\mu M$ and the observed structure–activity relationships seem to indicate specific interactions with a different binding site. A specific binding to the benzodiazepine receptor of freeze-dried rat cortex preparations, indicated by an inhibition of the $[^3H]$flunitrazepam binding, was not observed for the kavalactones. The radioreceptor assay was verified by an in-process procedure with an IC_{50} value of 9.8 nM for diazepam (Boonen and Haberlein, 1998). A novel new technique employing fluorescence correlation spectroscopy has confirmed specific interactions between a tetramethylrhodamine-labeled kavain derivative and human cortical neurons. Human cortical neurons were incubated with 1 nM of the dye-labeled kavain derivative. A total binding of 0.55 nM was found after an incubation period of 60 minutes. Fifty percent of the total binding was specifically displaced in the presence of 1 μM non-labeled (+)-kavain. Evidence for these specific interactions was verified by a saturation experiment. Both the non-linear Scatchard plot and the n value of 1.58 ± 0.07 in the sigmoid Hill plot indicated binding sites with different binding affinities (Boonen *et al.*, 2000).

Regional differences in the binding of kavalactones to $GABA_A$ receptors were studied using membrane fractions obtained from various target brain centers and the $GABA_A$ receptor antagonist [^{3}H] muscimol. Kavalactone enriched kava extracts, with final kavalactone concentrations ranging between 10 μM and 1 mM, augmented specific [^{3}H] muscimol binding to about 358% in the hippocampus, 300% in the amygdala, and 273% in the medulla oblongata ($P < 0.01$). Minimal stimulation was observed in the cerebellum followed by the frontal cortex (Figure 6.5). Similar concentrations of individual kavalactones were effective in the brain areas investigated, exhibiting IC_{50} values between 200 and 300 μM. Scatchard analysis revealed that the observed effects of kavalactones were due to an increase in the number of binding sites (B_{max}), rather than to a change in receptor-binding affinity (Jussofie *et al.*, 1994).

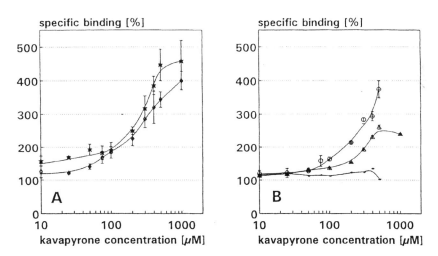

Figure 6.5 Concentration-dependence of the modulation of [^{3}H]muscimol binding to membrane fractions from different brain regions of ovariectomized rats in the presence of various concentrations of kava. The specific muscimol binding assessed in the absence of the kava extract was set at 100%. A. Two brain regions: ∗, hippocampus; ▲, amygdala. B. Three brain regions: ○, medulla; △, frontal cortex; ●, cerebellum. The cerebellum data are the mean of triplicate and two separate experiments; all other points are derived from three independent experiments. Reprinted from Jussofie *et al.* (1994) Kavapyrone enriched extract from *Piper methysticum* as a modulator of the GABA binding site in different regions of rat brain. *Psychopharmacology*, 116, 469–474, figure 2AB, with permission from Springer-Verlag.

Thus, strong evidence for the involvement of a GABAergic mechanism of pharmaco-logically relevant action by the kavalactones has been provided by the excellent correlation between $GABA_A$ receptor modulation elicited by kavalactones and their pharmacological potency. However, some discrepancies have been reported, for instance, Davies *et al.* (1992) found no binding of the lactones to rat forebrain $GABA_B$ receptors, and only weak activity at $GABA_A$ receptors. On the other hand, Holm *et al.* (1991) reported that limbic structures, especially the amygdala, were the main sites of action of kavalac-tones, and hence may explain the promotion of sleep by kava. These observations are supported by the fact noted above that these compounds show significant binding to $GABA_A$ receptors in the hippocampus and the amygdala, and minimal stimulation of the cerebellum and the frontal cortex (Jussofie *et al.*, 1994).

Furthermore, kavain (5–40 µM) and dihydromethysticin (10–40 µM) reversibly reduced the frequency of field potentials in the CA1 and CA3 areas in hippocampal slice preparations of guinea pigs, induced by activation of NMDA receptors and voltage-dependent Ca^{2+} channels (Walden *et al.*, 1997). These workers also found that kavalactones enhanced the anxiolytic effects of the $5HT_{1A}$ agonist ipsapirone, as evaluated by their effects on hippocampal field potentials. The most likely explanation for the brain regional specificity in kavalactone sensitivity of $GABA_A$ receptors is the existence of multiple $GABA_A$ receptor subtype genes that vary in brain regional expression (Olsen and Tobin, 1990). This conclusion is consistent with other findings which show brain regional differences in responses to benzodiazepines, bicuculline, and steroids (Massottti *et al.*, 1991; Sapp *et al.*, 1992; Jussofie, 1993).

Effects on monoamine uptake carriers

In light of the ability of kava to counteract fatigue, alleviate anxiety, and elicit contentment (Singh, 1992), studies were done to ascertain whether kavalactones could elevate CNS levels of monoamines which are involved in the pathophysiology of depression and anxiety by blocking their neuronal uptake (Seitz *et al.*, 1997a). The actions of the natural compounds (+)-kavain and (+)-methysticin, and the synthetic racemate (±)-kavain, were tested on *in vitro* uptake of the monoamines [^{3}H]-noradrenaline, and [^{3}H]-serotonin in synaptosomes prepared from the cerebral cortex and the hippocampus of rats. The monoamine uptake assay was verified by an in-process procedure using desipramine, a selective noradrenaline uptake inhibitor, which blocked [^{3}H]-noradrenaline uptake with a K_i value of 0.78 nM, and fluoxetine, a selective serotonin reuptake inhibitor, which blocked [^{3}H]-serotonin uptake with a K_i value of 402 nM. (±)-Kavain and (+)-kavain were less potent than desipramine and fluoxetine, and significant inhibition of [^{3}H]-noradrenaline uptake was only seen at concentrations above 10 µM. At the maximal concentration of 400 µM, the [^{3}H]-noradrenaline uptake was reduced almost equally by (±)-kavain and (+)-kavain to 70–80 % of control. The K_i values were in the same range and amounted to 48.7 µM and 59.6 µM, respectively. (+)-Methysticin was not as potent as (±)-kavain or (+)-kavain. At the maximal concentration of 400 µM, (+)-methysticin inhibited the [^{3}H]-noradrenaline uptake by only 45% of control. Despite their actions on [^{3}H]-noradrenaline uptake, the tested kavalactones were completely ineffective in concen-trations up to 100 µM which effectively blocked [^{3}H]-serotonin uptake, suggesting different affinities of the compounds for the [^{3}H]-serotonin and [^{3}H]-noradrenaline uptake carriers (Seitz *et al.*, 1997a).

Effects on neurotransmitters

In vivo methods were used to determine the effects of (+)-dihydromethysticin on striatal and cortical tissue concentrations of the neurotransmitters dopamine and serotonin, their respective metabolites 3,4-dihydroxyphenylacetic acid (DOPAC) and 5-hydroxy-indoleacetic acid (5-HIAA), as well as on dopamine and serotonin turnover. Additionally, rats were fed with a (±)-kavain-containing food (0.48 g/kg food) over a period of 78 days in order to evaluate the influence of chronic treatment with kavalactones on neurotransmitter levels. The study demonstrated that neither (+)-dihydromethysticin (100 mg/kg) in a single high dose, nor (±)-kavain chronically administered, significantly altered the striatal and cortical tissue levels or the turnover of dopamine or serotonin in rats ($P < 0.05$). However, a smaller weight gain in the (±)-kavain treated rats compared to the control group was found, even though both groups consumed nearly the same amount of food ($P < 0.05$) (Boonen *et al.*, 1998).

On the other hand, the microdialysis technique produced contrasting effects of kava extract and individual kavalactones on neurotransmitter levels in the nucleus accumbens of intact rats. After application of a kava extract (120 mg/kg ip), increased levels of dopamine were found. (±)-Kavain administered at low doses (30 mg/kg ip) induced a decrease in dopamine levels ($P < 0.002$), while at higher doses (120 mg/kg ip) there was either a small increase or no change in dopamine and the dopamine metabolite, homovanillic acid (HVA) concentrations, but a large increase in DOPAC. Yangonin (120 mg/kg ip) decreased dopamine levels below the detection limit ($P < 0.013$) while desmethoxyyangonin (120 mg/kg ip) caused an increase ($P < 0.034$). Dihydrokavain, methysticin, and dihydromethysticin did not produce any significant change in dopamine, DOPAC, or HVA levels ($P > 0.03$). (±)-Kavain (60 mg/kg ip) induced a decrease in 5-HT and 5-HIAA levels but the changes were not significant. Some of the other kavalactones also affected 5-HT levels as well, but the effects were not consistent and showed great variability between the different kavalactones (Sällström Baum *et al.*, 1998).

Pharmacokinetic–Pharmacodynamic Considerations

Despite the wide spectrum of pharmacological activities associated with the kavalactones and the number of compounds they represent, the present knowledge concerning them indicates that there are only slight differences in their mechanisms of action. Thus, the major differences distinguishing them appear to be in the pharmacokinetic properties of the individual compounds (Kretzschmar, 1995) and, if the kava extract is involved, their relative proportions. In general, the kavalactones, especially when present in the resin or lipid soluble form, are readily absorbed by the gastrointestinal tract and are bioavailable to the CNS. Furthermore, there is evidence to indicate that mixtures of kavalactones improve the bioavailability of individual lactones, as discussed below.

Rasmussen *et al.* (1979) attempted to measure by gas chromatography the n-octanol-water partition coefficients of the major kava lactones and found that these compounds could not be detected in the aqueous phase. Since the bulk of the earlier pharmacological work had concentrated on the water-soluble lactones, Buckley *et al.* (1979) investigated the biological activity of the water-soluble fractions of kava obtained by steam distillation. They found that the fractions so obtained contained biologically active materials that were relatively free of any lactones. These materials suppressed spontaneous activity in test animals and at higher doses led to muscular relaxation previously seen with the lactones. In addition, one of the two fractions exhibited an anti-serotonin activity similar to that of dihydromethysticin. Thus the composition and pharmacological activity may not be coincident for an aqueous kava extract and kava resin obtained by lipid extraction from the same raw material.

Keledjian *et al*. (1988) have measured the rate of uptake into mouse brain tissue of kavain, dihydrokavain, yangonin, and desmethoxyyangonin after their ip injection at a dose level of 100 mg/kg. Maximal brain concentrations of kavain and dihydrokavain occurred 5 minutes after administration. This rapid uptake is in accordance with the high lipid solubility of these compounds. These results are consistent with the observation by Meyer (1979) that the peak effect of the two compounds in protecting mice from maximal electroshock seizure occurred 10 minutes after their injection. For the other two lactones, desmethoxyyangonin and yangonin, the maximal brain concentrations were much lower and the time course followed a more diffuse profile after similar treatment. Meyer (1979) established that these two lactones possessed weak central nervous activity after a similar experimental protocol. Thus, the brain concentrations correlated well with the centrally mediated pharmacological actions exhibited by all four compounds.

Five minutes after ip injection in mice of single doses of individual kavalactones at 100 mg/kg, the maximal brain concentrations of the major lactones (μg/g wet brain tissue weight) were kavain (29.3±0.8), dihydrokavain (64.7±13.1), desmethoxyyangonin (10.4±1.5), and yangonin (1.2±0.3). After administration of the kava resin at 120 mg/kg (equivalent to 23 mg dihydrokavain, 44 mg kavain, 16 mg desmethoxyyangonin, and 18 mg yangonin), cerebral concentrations for kavain and yangonin were 27.8 and 4.6 μg/g wet brain tissue weight, respectively. In comparison to pure, single kavalactones, the administration of the extract increased the bioavailability of kavain two-fold and yangonin more than twenty-fold. The bioavailability of dihydrokavain and desmethoxyyangonin, however, was similar whether administered singly or as part of the rhizome extract (Keledjian *et al*., 1988). Clearly this finding supports the observation that a synergistic uptake effect operated in the animal studies when kava resin was compared with some of its individual constituents acting singly (Klohs *et al*., 1959; Kretzschmar *et al*., 1968). Meyer (1979) also reported that the activity of yangonin after ip application in preventing mice from maximal electroshock seizure was markedly increased when given in combination with other kavalactones. Thus, the synergism in pharmacological activity appears to be due to potentiation of uptake into the brain when the compounds are administered together rather than separately. The mechanism by which this occurs remains unclear. But in view of their high lipid solubility, plasma protein binding may be a significant factor, with competition for binding sites raising the free plasma lactone concentrations.

In an effort to develop a new special kava formulation from extracts of the kava rhizome, pharmacokinetic studies were conducted in mice and rats (Biber *et al*., 1992). After an oral dose of 100 mg/kg of the extract, the kavalactones reached maximum plasma levels of 0.3–0.9 μg/ml after 30 minutes. With 100 mg/kg of the test formulation given orally to mice and rats, bioavailability was clearly increased, the maximum plasma levels reaching 1.7–2.5 μg/ml of kavain, dihydrokavain, methysticin, and dihydomethysticin, and 0.3 μg/ml of yangonin after 30 minutes. The change in kavalactone levels in the brain was parallel to that in the plasma, and showed a peak concentration of 1.1–2.0 μg/g wet brain tissue weight. The elimination half-life of the kavalactones in mouse plasma and brain tissue was one hour and even longer in the rat. Thus, the bioavailability of kavalactones was increased by a factor of up to ten through the optimization of the galenical formulation (Biber *et al.*, 1992). In humans, a single oral dose of 200 mg (±)-kavain resulted in a maximum plasma concentration of 18 μg/ml. A distribution half-life of 3–5 hours and an elimination half-life of 9 hours were determined (Neuronika®, 1989).

More recently, a comparison was made of the oral bioavailability in mice and dogs of a formulation prepared from a kava extract (WS 1490, containing 70% kavalactones), with the extract itself and the pure compound (+)-kavain. In both species, bioavailability increased in the order, pure compound, extract, and extract formulation. The data confirm the above findings on the synergistic absorption and uptake of kavalactones, and indicate that clinical data from one preparation or formulation cannot simply be transferred to other formulations without appropriate biopharmaceutical characterization (Biber *et al.*, 2000).

The standardization procedure for the kavalactones in pharmaceutical preparations appear to have an important effect on the final results obtained. According to Gaedcke (2000), previous quantitation of the compounds was done by TLC, and the German Commission E monograph recommended daily dose of 60–120 mg of kavalactones was based on TLC values. Since 1980, HPLC techniques have been available for this purpose, and are now considered to be more accurate. It has been shown that 60 to 120 mg of kavalactones measured by the TLC method are equivalent to about 95 to 190 mg of kavalactones measured by HPLC. Furthermore, because of the highly lipophilic nature of the kavalactones, dry extracts are produced by adding large amounts of excipients. In the so-called "purified extracts," the level of resinous lipophilic constituents are reduced from the conventional "total extracts." Thus, in the manufacture of the final dosage form, such as tablets or capsules, the selection of the analytical procedure and the excipients used can have profound impact on the resulting composition and biopharmaceutical properties of the products. The urgent necessity to develop a uniform standardization procedure for kavalactones has been addressed by others. Janeczko and Podolak (2000) have proposed what they claim is a "practical, easy and quick test for routine control of the roots and commercial preparations of kava–kava," in which TLC is combined with the computer programme "Chroma." The extracts are chromatographed on TLC plates in a solvent system containing a dioxan-hexane (3:7) mixture and kavalactones are visualized by 25% methanol-H_2SO_4. The spots are scanned and transformed into graphic signals, the peak areas of which are then calculated.

Toxicology

There are many reports in the historical and ethnographic literature on the adverse effects of kava beverage consumption, and some of this material is discussed in detail elsewhere in this volume. In this section, the more recent and scientific reports will be considered.

In acute toxicity studies, the LD_{50} of kava resin given by ip injection to mice, rats, and rabbits ranged from 300 to 400 mg/kg. With oral administration, the LD_{50} in mice was 920 mg/kg for dihydrokavain and 1050 mg/kg for dihydromethysticin (Meyer, 1962). However, doses of 50 mg/kg of dihydromethysticin, administered three times a week for three months to rats, produced no evidence of chronic toxicity (Meyer, 1966).

Kava resin administered orally to mice produced no loss of righting reflex in doses less than 200 mg/kg. Doses between 250 and 300 mg/kg produced short-term loss of righting reflex in four of eight mice, while consistent loss of the righting reflex was seen at 350 mg/kg. Sleeping times increased as the dose was raised to 600 mg/kg, at which point one of six mice died. Doses of 700 mg/kg or higher of kava resin produced lethality in more than 50% of the mice tested (Jamieson and Duffield, 1990a).

In a study on medical students, Frater (1958) found that the subjects, on chewing on 1.5 oz (43 g) of kava root or drinking 2 liters of a kava beverage (composition not given) over 2 hours, felt lethargic, were unable to concentrate on their studies, and felt weak at the knees, their eyes were watery and slightly bloodshot, with enlarged pupils which reacted slowly to light. However, there was no effect on their speech and reasoning or ability to walk in a straight line or run up stairs two at a time. As noted earlier, enlarged pupil diameter as well as reduced distance vision leading to disturbances in oculomotor balance were observed by Garner and Klinger (1985) in individuals who drank a moderate amount of kava. Earlier, Steinmetz (1960) suggested that consumption of too much kava by humans manifests as difficulty in walking, enlarged pupils slow to react to light, and sleepiness. However, he also noted that higher centers of mental function remain relatively undisturbed.

Anecdotal accounts of kava causing nausea, vomiting, and headache can be found in the literature. However, most of the subjects were naïve drinkers, and experienced users of the beverage do not have the same experience. Kava cultivars high in dihydrokavain and dihydromethysticin are more likely to cause nausea and headache (Lebot and Lévesque, 1989).

In a report from Germany, four patients who took kava in a dose of 100 mg of standardized kava extract (Laitan®, W. Schwabe, Germany) for anxiety as prescribed by their physician, developed clinical symptoms suggestive of central dopaminergic antagonism. These symptoms manifested as involuntary oral and lingual dyskinesia, involuntary neck extension with forceful upward deviation of eyes, rotation of the head to the right, and painful twisting movement of the trunk. These complications were reversed spontaneously by discontinuing kava use or by anticholinergic anti-Parkinson drugs like biperiden (Schelosky *et al.*, 1995).

Siegers (1993) has noted a lack of negative impact on driving ability after kava consumption but, unfortunately, details on the dosage were not provided. However, overconsumption and subsequent operation of a motor vehicle resulted in arrest and conviction of a Utah (USA) motorist for "driving under the influence of kava." The man told police he had consumed about 16 cups of the beverage, his usual dose being one or two (Swensen, 1996).

Cutaneous effects

The effect of chronic kava drinking on the skin has been mentioned in many historical and ethnographic reports (Beechey, 1831; Thomson, 1908; Titcomb, 1948), and is invoked in several legends from the Pacific (see Chapter 2). The lesion in question, called *kani* or *kanikani* in Fijian, requires regular, almost daily, consumption of kava before it appears, and takes from a few months to a year or more to develop. The skin becomes dry, yellowish, and covered with scales, especially the palms of the hand, the soles of the feet, the forearms, back and shins (Figure 6.6). However, there have been only a few reported attempts to understand the pathophysiological basis for it and to search for a cure. Proposed causes include accumulation of plant pigments (Shulgin,

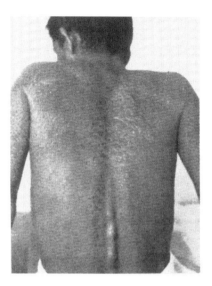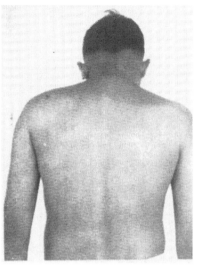

Figure 6.6 Left: A case of the skin lesion, kava dermopathy, on the back of a chronic kava drinker. Right: The same subject six months after a reduction in kava consumption and a balanced diet. Reprinted from Singh (1992) Kava: an overview. *Journal of Ethnopharmacology*, 7, 13–45, with permission from Elsevier Science.

1973) or kavalactones (Siegel, 1976), chronic allergic dermatitis (Lebot and Cabalion, 1988), reduction in glandular secretions (Davidson, 1899), persistent light reaction, and a pellagra-like dermatosis (Frater, 1958). Frater came to the tentative conclusion that kani was caused through interference by kava of the normal uptake and assimilation of some members of the group B vitamins. The condition could be reversed, even in the most serious cases, by a reduction in kava consumption and a balanced diet (Figure 6.6). On prolonged use and in high doses of dihydromethysticin (300–800 mg/day) a high percentage of subjects developed exfoliative dermatitis, characterized by dry scaly skin similar to kava dermopathy (Keller and Klohs, 1963).

Because of its resemblance to pellagra, kava dermopathy was also believed to be due to a deficiency of the vitamin niacin (or nicotinamide), but this theory has since been disproved (Ruze, 1990). In her study, Ruze selected 29 male Tongan kava drinkers, all of whom showed the characteristic skin lesions. Fifteen of these individuals were randomized to receive a dose of niacin, while the remaining 14 received a placebo containing no active ingredient. After three weeks, clinical improvement was observed in five members from each group. These finding led Ruze to conclude that niacin vitamin deficiency was not responsible for the skin condition since treatment with the vitamin did not produce an effect significantly different from control. The lesion is now thought to be related to interference with cholesterol metabolism, a theory supported by a study on heavy kava usage in an Australian Aboriginal community (Mathews *et al.*, 1988; Norton and Ruze, 1994).

Jappe *et al.* (1998) reported two clinical cases of drug-induced eruption in sebaceous gland-rich areas, induced by two to three weeks of systemic kava therapy. In the first case, a 70-year old man was also taking multiple drugs, including nitrofurantoin, allopurinol, spironolactone, furosemide, yohimbine, and mesterolone. After sunlight exposure for several hours, itching occurred, followed by erythematous, infiltrated plaques on the ventral and dorsal thorax and the face. Laboratory tests excluded lupus erythematosus, which occasionally may be induced by nitrofurantoin, allopurinol, spironolactone, or furosemide, as well as photodermatosis related to yohimbine. However, a standardized diagnostic allergy test revealed significant proliferation of peripheral blood lymphocytes with kava extract. The second patient, after three weeks of systemic therapy with kava extract, was seen with papules and plaques on the face and later on her dorsal and ventral thorax and arms. She also had a strongly positive patch test to kava extract after 24 hours in contrast to negative results in a control group of 20 adults. A hematogenous allergic contact dermatitis after oral administration of kava extract has also been described by Süss and Lehmann (1996).

A 47 year old woman, two weeks after taking an unknown amount of kava for anxiety, noticed a rash in the neck area that later involved the back, upper extremities, and face, and also worsening proximal muscle weakness. Her creatine kinase level was elevated and an electromyogram showed a myopathic pattern. Skin and muscle biopsy samples showed changes consistent with dermatomyositis. The patient improved with prednisone and discontinuation of kava (Guro-Razuman *et al.*, 1999).

Hepatotoxicity

A total of about 40 clinical cases of liver damage which may be connected with kava use have recently been reported from Europe, mainly Germany and Switzerland, and also from North America, Australia, and New Zealand (Strahl *et al.*, 1998; Brunner, 2000: Hellwig, 2000; Stoller, 2000; Brauer *et al.*, 2001; Escher *et al.*, 2001; Kraft *et al.*, 2001; Russmann *et al.*, 2001; Sass *et al.*, 2001; Schmidt, 2001). In addition to skin eruptions, headaches, lightheadedness, cases of extrapyramidal disorders, speech, vision, and accommodation problems were also reported. In some patients, jaundice arose with considerable increases in bilirubin and transaminases, and some elevation of alkaline phosphatases, while an additional decrease in Quick value (which is an indicator of blood clotting time) to below 50% was observed in three of these patients. Hepatic necrosis in a few patients was serious enough to warrant liver transplantation which was carried out successfully. However, it appears that the extracts were prepared using organic solvents, such as acetone and ethanol, which are known to be hepatotoxins themselves, or which might have extracted other toxic constituents. These and other possibilities are further discussed in Chapter 7. Presently, there are no experimental data in the literature to indicate a causal linkage between the kavalactones and hepatotoxicity.

Interactions with other substances

In mice and rabbits, lipid soluble kava extract and some kavalactones significantly prolonged barbiturate-induced sleeping time and protected against the lethal effects of strychnine (Klohs *et al.*, 1959; Meyer, 1962; Hänsel, 1968). Also, the kava extract and ethanol prolonged each others sleeping time, so that a sub-hypnotic dose of one potentiated a minimally effective hypnotic dose of the other (Jamieson and Duffield, 1990b,c). For instance, subhypnotic doses of ethanol (2 and 3 g/kg ip) prolonged the sleeping time of 350 mg/kg po of kava resin from 13.8 ± 3.4 minutes to 60.3 ± 10.9 minutes and 143.5 ± 14.9 minutes, respectively. A dose of 600 mg/kg of kava resin alone was required to cause a sleeping time of 148 ± 34.1 minutes. Conversely, subhypnotic doses of kava resin of 200 and 300 mg/kg ip increased the sleeping time of 3.5 g/kg ethanol from 35.5 ± 7.4 minutes to 94.3 ± 5.3 minutes and 116.3 ± 10.8 minutes, respectively. Furthermore, 2 mg/kg of ethanol, when combined with a moderately effective dose of kava extract (450 mg/kg), was lethal in 60% of mice tested. This possible interaction between kava and ethanol has important social and clinical implications as, in contrast to traditional usage, kava is now often taken in conjunction with alcoholic beverages.

In a placebo-controlled, randomized double-blind trial, there were no significant negative effects on safety related performance from a recommended dose of 3×100 mg/ day of standardized kava extract in humans with blood alcohol concentration of 0.05% (Herberg, 1993). However, Foo and Lemon (1997) found that a subthreshold dosage of kava (1 g/kg) significantly worsened ($P < 0.05$) alcohol-induced (BAC 0.05–0.15%) impairment in the ratings on five subjective measures of sedation, cognition, coordination, intoxication, and willingness to drive, and four performance tests of physical and mental coordination and function.

In the only reported clinical case of interaction involving kava and prescription medications, a 54-year old man suffered from a coma when he added kava to alprazolam, cimetidine, and terazosin he was already taking (Almeida and Grimsley, 1996). His vital signs and results of laboratory studies were normal. His alcohol level was negative, and a drug screen was positive for benzodiazepines. He became more alert after several hours and denied overdosing on the kava or alprazolam. This incident was probably due to an interaction on GABAergic or benzodiazepine receptors between kava, as kavalactones actively bind to GABAergic receptors, and alprazolam.

Sports related deaths among Australian Aboriginal athletes prompted a study to determine the incidence of sudden cardiac death due to ischemic heart disease (IHD) (Young *et al.*, 1999). In a sample size of eight football players, all of whom suffered from IHD, four of the players had drunk large amounts of alcohol or kava (some possibly both) the evening before the game. Both of these drinks have diuretic properties, which may contribute to dehydration and hemoconcentration, thus increasing the cardiovascular stress of exercise, especially in the absence of adequate fluid replacement. An association between kava use and sudden cardiac death has previously been suggested (Mathews *et al.*, 1988) and may be supported by the present study.

In a survey on the health status of 39 kava users and 34 non-users in a coastal Aboriginal community in Arnhem Land in northern Australia, Mathews *et al.* (1988) found that very heavy users (average consumption of 440 g/week) were 20% underweight, and more likely to complain of general poor health and various medical disorders. For instance, they presented the typical scaly skin rash of kava dermopathy, shortness of breath, slightly increased patellar reflexes, underweight, incoordination, possibly pulmonary hypertension, red eyes, reduced plasma protein, albumin, urea, and bilirubin, decreased platelet and lymphocyte count, poorly acidified urine, more likely to show hematuria, and other alterations in renal and liver function. On the basis of the above observations, these workers recommended urgent social action to improve the health in Aboriginal communities by reducing kava consumption and improving nutritional status of kava users. However, these findings have been widely challenged, as Aboriginal health is considered to be generally worse than for other Australian groups and the survey subjects may already have been in poor health before taking up kava (Devanesen *et al.*, 1986), or may have been using other stimulants like alcohol and nicotine at the same time and not revealing this to the clinical study (Douglas, 1988; Lebot *et al.*, 1997).

Tolerance and addiction potential

The overindulgence of kava by some Pacific islanders and Australian Aborigines may be seen as suggestive of tolerance. Because it is believed that a strong correlation exists between tolerance and drug dependence, Duffield and Jamieson (1991) investigated the development of tolerance to kava in mice. They observed a very rapidly developing tolerance to the aqueous lactone-free extract, but not with the lipid soluble resin fraction. As tolerance was evident at the first test period it was assumed to be physiological tolerance, although some partial tolerance was noted with high doses of the kava resin administered over a three-week period. However, there is no evidence in the literature to suggest that kava use leads to addiction or dependency (Lebot and Lévesque, 1989).

Mutagenicity and teratogenicity

No scientific studies or reports on the mutagenicity or teratogenicity were found in the literature. However, native populations throughout the Pacific have been using kava for generations without any apparent side-effects of these types.

Carcinogenicity

As with mutagenicity and teratogenicity, no carcinogenic effects have been reported for kava in the literature. In fact recent reports suggest that a correlation might exist between kava consumption and the low incidence of cancer in many of the South Pacific countries (Steiner, 2000). Data were compiled from cancer incidence studies which were completed in the 1980s for the following Pacific Islands: Fiji (Singh *et al.*, 1986), Vanuatu (Paksoy *et al.*, 1990), Western Samoa (Paksoy *et al.*, 1991), Micronesia (Henderson *et al.*, 1995), and New Caledonia (Thevenot *et al.*, 1986). Hawaii (Hawaiians), New Zealand (Maoris) and USA (Los Angeles) (Muir *et al.*, 1987) were also included in the comparative study. Los Angeles Caucasians served as a reference population which was non-kava consuming and was not ethnically related to the Oceanic people. The Hawaiians and the New Zealand Maoris are Polynesians who do not use kava at the present time. For the same period of time, local kava consumption statistics were also available (Lebot *et al.*, 1997).

The data showed that New Zealand, Hawaii and Los Angeles had the highest age-standardized cancer incidence (307–322 per 100,000 male population) and the lowest annual kava consumption (0 kg per person) followed by New Caledonia (182; 0.6), Micronesia (132; 1.4), Western Samoa (90.2; 2.2), Fiji (75; 2.8), and finally Vanuatu which had the lowest cancer incidence and the highest kava consumption (71; 6.7). However, if kava does reduce the incidence of cancer, it may not be the sole chemoprotective agent responsible. Other factors which may impact the findings need to be considered before any definitive, even tentative conclusions can be made. These factors include genetics and related susceptibility to carcinogenic factors, and those which may be associated to the environment, diet, and lifestyle, in particular, exposure to short wavelength radiation, chemical carcinogens, tobacco, and microbial infection.

Precautions and contraindications

Studies in animals and humans suggest that kava should be avoided or used with caution in pregnancy, by nursing mothers, and patients suffering from Parkinson's disease, muscle diseases, and endogenous depression (Blumenthal *et al.*, 1998). Kava acts on a number of receptors, including GABAergic, serotonergic, dopaminergic, and sodium ion channels, and therefore may possibly interact with pharmaceuticals which act at these receptors (Jussofie *et al.*, 1994; Schelosky *et al.*, 1995). Thus, kava should not be used with selective serotonin reuptake inhibitors, tricyclic antidepressants, barbiturates, benzodiazepines, alcohol, and various antipsychotics, or should be used under a physician's supervision. Even when administered in its prescribed dosages, kava may affect motor reflexes and impair judgment for driving or operating heavy machinery (Blumenthal *et al.*, 1998).

References

Almeida, J. and Grimsley, E. (1996) Coma from the health food store. Interaction between kava and alprazolam. *Annals of Internal Medicine*, 125(1), 940–941.

Backhauss, C. and Krieglstein, J. (1992a) Extract of kava (*Piper methysticum*) and its methysticin constituents protect brain tissue against ischemic damage in rodents. *European Journal of Pharmacology*, 215, 265–269.

Backhauss, C. and Krieglstein, J. (1992b) Neuroprotective activity of kava extract (*Piper methysticum*) and its methysticin constituents *in vivo* and *in vitro*. In J. Krieglstein and H. Oberpichler-Schwenk (eds), *Pharmacology of Cerebral Ischemia*, Wissenschftliche Verlagsgellschaft mBH, Stuttgart, pp. 501–507.

Beechey, F.W. (1831) *Narrative of a Voyage to the Pacific and Bering's Strait*, Colburn and Bentley, London. Reprinted 1968, 2 vols. N. Israel, Amsterdam, vol. 2, pp. 120–122.

Benveniste, H.J., Drejer, J., Schouboe, A. and Diemer, N.H. (1984) Elevation of the extracellular concentrations of glutamate and aspartate in rat hippocampus during transient cerebral ischemia monitored by intracerebral microdialysis. *Journal of Neurochemistry*, 43, 1369.

Biber, A., Nöldner, M. and Schlegelmilch, R. (1992) Development of a formulation of Kava extract through pharmacokinetic experiments in animals. *Naunyn Schmiedeberg's Archives of Pharmacology*, 345 *(Suppl.)*, R24.

Biber, A., Oschmann, R., Lang, F., Nöldner, M. and Chatterjee, S.S. (2000) Pharmacokinetic and biopharmaceutical aspects of kavalactones and kava-kava extract containing formulations. *Phytomedicine*, 7(Suppl. II), 27–28.

Bliss, T.V.P. and Collingridge, G.L. (1993) A synaptic model of memory: long-term potentiation in the hippocampus. *Nature*, 361, 31–39.

Blumenthal, M., Busse, W., Goldberg, A., Gruenwald, J., Hall, T., Riggins, C. and Rister, R. (1998) *The Complete German Commission E Monographs. Therapeutic Guide to Herbal Medicine*, American Botanical Council, Austin, Texas.

Boonen, G. and Häberlein, H. (1998) Influence of genuine kavapyrone enantiomers on the $GABA_A$ binding site. *Planta Medica*, 64, 504–506.

Boonen, G., Ferger, B., Kuschinsky, K. and Häberlein H. (1998) *In vivo* effects of the kavapyrones (+)-dihydromethysticin and (±)-kavain on dopamine, 3,4-dihydroxyphenylacetic acid, serotonin and 5-hydroxyindoleacetic acid levels in striatal and cortical brain regions. *Planta Medica*, 64, 507–510.

Boonen, G., Pramanik, A., Rigler. R. and Häberlein, H. (2000) Evidence for specific interactions between kavain and human cortical neurons monitored by fluorescence correlation spectroscopy. *Planta Medica*, 66, 7–10.

Borsche, W. and Blount, B.K. (1933) Untersuchungen über die Bestandteile der Kawawurzel. XIII (vörlauf.) Mitteil, Über einige neue Stoffe aus technischem Kawaharz. *Chemische Berichte*, 66, 803–806.

Brauer, R.B., Pfab, R. and Becker, K. (2002) Fulminantes Leberversagen nach Einnahme des Pflanzlichen Heilmittels Kava-Kava [in German]. *Zeitschrift fur Gastroenterologie*, 39, 491(P30).

Brüggemann, F. and Meyer, H.J. (1963) Die analgetische Wirkung der Kawa-Inhaltsstoffe Dihydrokawain und Dihydromethysticin. *Arzneimittelforschung*, 13, 407–409.

Brunner, U. (2000) Leberschäden durch Kava-Extrakte. *Pharmazie*, 29, 55.

Buchsbaum, M.S., Hazlett, E., Sicotte, N., Stein, M., Wu, J. and Zetin, M. (1985) Topographic EEG changes with benzodiazepine administration in generalized anxiety disorder. *Biological Psychiatry*, 20, 832–842.

Buckley, J.P., Furgiuele, A.R. and O'Hara, M.J. (1979) Pharmacology of kava. In D.H. Efron, B. Holmstedt, and N.S. Kline (eds), *Ethnopharmacologic Search for Psychoactive Drugs*, Raven Press, New York, pp. 141–151.

Davidson, C. (1899) Hawaiian medicine. *Medical Age*, May 5, 1899, pp. 373–381. Quoted in Norton and Ruze (1994).

Davies, L.P., Drew, C.A., Duffield, P., Johnston, G.A.R. and Jamieson, D.D. (1992) Kavapyrones and resin: Studies on $GABA_A$, $GABA_B$ and benzodiazepine binding sites in rodent brain. *Pharmacology and Toxicology*, 71, 120–126.

Devanesen, D., Furber, M. and Hampton, D. (1986) *Health Indicators in the Northern Territory*, Northern Territory Department of Health, Darwin, NT.

Douglas, W. (1988) The effects of heavy usage of kava on physical health. *Medical Journal of Australia*, 149, 341–342.

Duffield, A.M. and Jamieson, D.D. (1988) Chemistry and pharmacology of kava. In J. Prescott, G. McCall (eds), *Kava: Use and Abuse in Australia and the South Pacific*, National Drug and Alcohol Research Centre, University of New South Wales, Sydney, Monograph 5, pp. 1–12.

Duffield, P.H. and Jamieson, D.D. (1991) Development of tolerance to kava in mice. *Clinical and Experimental Pharmacology and Physiology* 18, 571–578.

Duffield, P.H., Jamieson, D.D. and Duffield, A.M. (1989a) Effect of aqueous and lipid-soluble extracts of kava on the conditioned avoidance response in rats. *Archives Internationales des Pharmacodynamie*, 301, 81–90.

Duffield, A.M., Jamieson, D.D., Lidgard, R.O., Duffield, P.H. and Bourne, D.J. (1989b) Identification of some human urinary metabolites of the intoxicating beverage kava. *Journal of Chromatography*, 475, 273–281.

Escher, M., Desmeules, J., Giostra, E. and Mentha, G. (2001) Hepatitis associated with kava, a herbal remedy for anxiety. *British Medical Journal*, 322 (7278), 139.

Ferger, B., Boonen, G., Häberlein, H. and Kuschinsky, K. (1998) *In vivo* microdialysis study of (±)-kavain on veratridine-induced glutamate release. *European Journal of Pharmacology*, 347, 211–214.

Foo, H. and Lemon, J. (1997) Acute effects of kava, alone or in combination with alcohol, on subjective measures of impairment and intoxication and on cognitive performance. *Drug and Alcohol Review*, 16(2), 147–155.

Frater, A.S. (1958) Medical aspects of *yaqona. Transactions and Proceedings of the Fiji Society*, 5(2), 31–39.

Friese, J. and Gleitz, J. (1998) Kavain, dihydrokavain and dihydromethysticin non-competitively inhibit the specific binding of [3H]-batrachotoxinin-A 20–α–benzoate to receptor site 2 of voltage-gated Na^+ channels. *Planta Medica*, 64, 458–459.

Gaedcke, F. (2000) Pharmaceutical characterization of kava-kava extracts and their formulations. *Phytomedicine*, 7(Suppl. II), 27.

Garner, L. and Klinger, J. (1985) Some visual effects caused by the beverage kava. *Journal of Ethnopharmacology*, 13, 307–311.

Gessner, B. and Cnota, P. (1994) Untersuchungen der Vigilanz nach Applikation von Kava-Extrakt, Diazepam oder Plazebo. *Zeitschrift fur Phytotherapie*, 15, 30–37.

Gleitz, J., Beile, A. and Peters, T. (1995) (±)-Kavain inhibits the veratridine-activated voltage-dependent Na$^+$-channels in synaptosomes prepared from rat cerebral cortex. *Neuropharmacology*, 343(9), 1133–1138.

Gleitz, J., Beile, A. and Peters, T. (1996d) (±)-Kavain inhibits the veratridine and KCl-induced increase in intracellular Ca^{2+} and glutamate-release of rat cerebrocortical synaptosomes. *Neuropharmacology*, 35(2), 179–186.

Gleitz, J., Beile, A., Wilkens, P., Ameri, A. and Peters, T. (1997) Antithrombotic action of the kava pyrone (+)-kavain prepared from *Piper methysticum* on human platelets. *Planta Medica*, 63, 27–30.

Gleitz, J., Gottner, N., Ameri, A. and Peters, T. (1996a) Kavain inhibits non-stereospecifically veratridine–activated Na$^+$-channels. *Planta Medica*, 62, 580–581.

Gleitz, J., Tosch, C., Beile A. and Peters, T. (1996c) The protective action of tetrodotoxin and (±)-kavain on anaerobic glycolysis, ATP content and intracellular Na$^+$ and Ca^{2+} of anoxic brain vesicles. *Neuropharmacology*, 35(12), 1743–1752.

Gleitz , J., Friese, J., Beile, A., Ameri, A. and Peters, T. (1996b) Anticonvulsive action of (±)-kavain estimated from its properties on stimulated synaptosomes and Na$^+$ channel receptor sites. *European Journal of Pharmacology*, 315, 89–97.

Gracza, L. and Ruff, P. (1980) Einfache Methode zur Trennung und quantitativen Bestimmung von Kawa-Laktonen durch Hochleistungs-Flüssigkeits-Chromatographie. *Journal of Chromatography*, 193, 486–490.

Guro-Razuman, A., Anand, P., Hu, Q. and Mir, R. (1999) Dermatomyositis-like illness following kava-kava ingestion. *Journal of Clinical Rheumatology*, 5(6), 342–345.

Hänsel, R. (1968) Characterization and physiological activity of some kava constituents. *Pacific Science*, 22, 293–312.

Hänsel, R. and Beiersdorff, H.U. (1959) Zur Kenttnis der Sedativen Prinzipien des Kava-Rhizoms. *Arzneimittelforschung*, 9, 581–585.

Heinze, H.J., Münte, T.F., Steitz, J. and Matzke, M. (1994) Pharmacopsychological effects of oxazepam and kava-extract in a visual search paradigm assessed with event-related potentials. *Pharmacopsychiatry*, 27, 224–230.

Hellwig, B. (2000) Lösen Kava-Kava–Präparate Leberschäden aus? *Deutsche Apotheker Zeitung*, 29, 43–48.

Henderson, B.E., Kolonel, L.N., Dworshy, R., Kerford, D., Mori, E. Singh, K., *et al.* (1995) *Cancer Incidence in the Islands of the Pacific*. National Cancer Institute Monograph, 69, 3–81.

Herberg, K.W. (1993) Effect of kava special extract WS 1490 combined with ethyl alcohol on safety-relevant performance parameters. Blutalkohol, 30(2), 96–105. (English abstract).

Herberg, K.W. (1996) Alltagssicherheit unter Kava-Extrakt, Bromazepam und deren Kombination. *Z. Allg. Med.*, 73, 973–977.

Hocart, A.M. (1929) *Lau Islands, Fiji*, Bulletin No. 62, Bernice P. Bishop Museum Press, Honolulu, pp. 59–70.

Hogg, S. (1996) A review of the validity and variability of the elevated plus-maze as an animal model of anxiety. *Pharmacology, Biochemistry, and Behavior*, 54, 21–30.

Holm, E., Staedt, U., Hepp, J., Kortsik, C., Behne, F., Kaske, A., *et al.* (1991) Untersuchungen zum Wirkungsprofil von D,L-Kavain. *Arzneimittelforschung*, 41(7), 673–683.

Jamieson, D.D. and Duffield, P.H. (1990a) The antinociceptive actions of kava components in mice. *Clinical and Experimental Pharmacology and Physiology*, 17, 495–508.

Jamieson, D.D. and Duffield, P.H. (1990b) Interaction of kava and ethanol in mice. *European Journal of Pharmacology*, 183, 559.

Jamieson, D.D. and Duffield, P.H. (1990c) Positive interaction of ethanol and kava resin in mice. *Clinical and Experimental Pharmacology and Physiology*, 17, 509–514.

Jamieson, D.D., Duffield, P.H., Cheng, D. and Duffield, A.M. (1989) Comparison of the central nervous system activity of the aqueous and lipid extract of kava (*Piper methysticum*). *Archives Internationales des Pharmacodynamie*, **301**, 66–80.

Janeczko, Z. and Podolak, I. (2000) Quantitative analysis of kavapyrones in kava-kava (*Piper methysticum* Forst.) with computer program "Chroma". *Phytomedicine*, 7(Suppl. II), 80.

Jappe, U., Francke, I., Reinhold, D. and Gollnick, H.P.M. (1998) Sebotropic drug reaction resulting from kava-kava extract therapy: a new entity? *Journal of the American Academy of Dermatology*, **38**, 104–106.

Johnson, D., Frauendorf, A., Stecker, K. and Stein, U. (1991) Neurophysiologisches Wirkprofil und Verträglichkeit von Kava-Extrakt WS 1490. *TW Neurol. Psychiat.*, **5**, 349–354.

Jussofie, A. (1993) Brain area specific differences in the effects of neuroactive steroids on the GABA$_A$ Receptor complexes following acute treatment with anaesthetically active steroids. *Acta Endocrinology*, **129**, 480–485.

Jussofie, A., Schmitz, A. and Hiemke, C. (1994) Kavapyrones enriched extract from *Piper methysticum* as modulator of the GABA binding site in different regions of rat brain. *Psychopharmacology*, **116**, 469–474.

Keledjian, J., Duffield, P.H., Jamieson, D.D., Lidgard, R.O. and Duffield, A.M. (1988) Uptake into mouse brain of four compounds present in the psychoactive beverage kava. *Journal of Pharmaceutical Sciences*, 77(12), 1003–1006.

Keller, F. and Klohs, M. (1963) A review of the chemistry and pharmacology of the constituents of *Piper methysticum*. *Lloydia*, 26(1), 1–15.

Klohs, M.W., Keller, F., Williams, E., Toekes, M.I. and Cronheim, G.E. (1959) A chemical and pharmacological investigation of *Piper methysticum* Forst. *Journal of Medicinal and Pharmaceutical Chemistry*, 1(1), 95–103.

Kraft, M., Spahn, T.W., Menzel, J., Senninger, N., Dietl, K.H., Herbst, H., *et al.* (2001) Fulminantes Leberversagen nach Einnahme des pflanzlichen Antidepressivums Kava-Kava [in German]. *Deutsche Medizinische Wochenschrift*, **126**, 970–972.

Kretzschmar, R. (1995) Pharmakologische Untersuchungen zur zentralnervösen Wirkung und zum Wirkungsmechanismus der Kava-Droge (Piper methysticum) und ihrer kristallinen Inhaltsstoffe. In D. Loew and N. Rietbrock (eds), *Phytopharmaka in Forschung und klinischer Anwendung*, Steinkopff-Verlag, Darmstadt, pp. 65–74.

Kretzschmar, R. and Meyer, H.J. (1969) Vergleichende Untersuchungen über die antikonvulsive Wirksamkeit der Pyronverbindungen aus *Piper methysticum* Forst. *Archives Internationales des Pharmacodynamie*, 177(2), 261–277.

Kretzschmar, R. and Teschendorf, H.J. (1974) Pharmakologische Untersuchungen zur sedativ-tranquilisierenden Wirkung des Rauschpfeffers (*Piper methysticum* Forst). *Chemiker. Z.*, **1**, 24–28.

Kretzschmar, R., Meyer. H.J. and Teschendorf, H.J. (1968) Yangonin-eine pharmakologisch wirksame Pyronverbindung aus *Piper methysticum* Forst. *Naunyn Schmiedeberg's Archives of Exoerimental Pathology and Pharmacology*, **260**(2), 159–160.

Kretzschmar, R., Meyer, J., Teschendorf, H.J. and Zöllner, B. (1969) Antagonistische Wirkung natürlicher 5,6-hydrierter Kawa-Pyrone auf die Strychninvergidtung und den experimentellen lokalen Tetanus. *Archives Internationales des Pharmacodynamie*, 182(2), 251–268.

Kretzschmar, R., Teschendorf, H.J., Ladous, A. and Ettehadieh, D. (1971) On the sedative action of the kava rhizome (*Piper methysticum*). *Acta Pharmacology and Toxicology*, **29**(Suppl. 4), 24–28.

Langosch, J.M., Normann, C., Schirrmacher, K., Berger, M. and Walden, J. (1998) The influence of (±)-kavain on population spikes and long-term potentiation in guinea pig hippocampal slices. *Comparative Biochemistry and Physiology*, **120**, 545–549.

Lebot, V. and Cabalion, P. (1988) *Kavas of Vanuatu: Cultivars of* Piper methysticum *Forst.*, Technical paper No. 195, South Pacific Commission, Noumea, pp 3–53.

Lebot, V. and Lévesque, J. (1989) The origin and distribution of kava (*Piper methysticum*). A phytochemical approach. *Allertonia*, 5(2), 223–281.

Lebot, V., Merlin, M. and Lindstrom, L. (1997) *Kava, the Pacific Elixir*, Healing Arts Press, Rochester VT.

Lemert, E.M. (1967) Secular use of kava in Tonga. *Quarterly Journal of Studies in Alcohol*, 28, 328–341.

Lewin, L. (1886) *Über* Piper methysticum *(Kawa)*, A. Hirschwald, Berlin.

Locher, C.P., Burch, M.T., Mower, H.F., Berestecky, Davis, H., Van Poel, B., Lasure, A., *et al.* (1995) Anti-microbial activity and anti-complement activity of extracts obtained from selected Hawaiian medicinal plants. *Journal of Ethnopharmacology*, 49, 23–32.

Magura, E.I., Kopanitsa, M.V., Gleitz, J., Peters, T. and Krishtal, O.A. (1997) Kava extract ingredients (+) methysticin and (±)-kavain inhibit voltage-operated Na^+ channels in rat CA1 hippocampal neurons. *Neuroscience*, 81(2), 345–351.

Martin, H.B., Stofer, D.S. and Eichinger, M.R. (2000) Kavain inhibits murine airway smooth muscle contraction. *Planta Medica*, 66, 601–606.

Martin, H.B., McCallum, M., Stofer, D.S. and Eichinger, M.R. (2002) Kavain attenuates vascular contractility through inhibition of calcium channels. *Planta Medica*, 68, 784–789.

Massottti, M., Schlichting, J.L., Antonacci, M.D., Giusti, P., Memo, M., Costa, E., *et al.* (1991) Gamma-aminobutyric acid: A receptor heterogeneity in rat central nervous system: studies with clonazepam and other benzodiazepine ligands. *Journal of Experimental Pharmacology and Therapeutics*, 256, 1154–1160.

Mathews, J.D., Riley, M.D., Fejo, L., Munoz, E., Milns, N.R., Gardner, I.D., *et al.* (1988) Effects of the heavy usage of kava on physical health: Summary of a pilot survey in an Aboriginal community. *Medical Journal of Australia*, 148, 548–555.

Meldrum, B.S., Evans, M., Griffiths, T. and Simon, R. (1985) Ischemic brain damage: The role of excitatory activity and of calcium entry. *British Journal of Anaesthesia*, 57, 44–51.

Meyer, H.J. (1962) Pharmakologie der wirksamen Prinzipien des Kawa-Rhizoms (*Piper methysticum* Forst). *Archives Internationales des Pharmacodynamie*, 138(3–4), 505–536.

Meyer, H.J. (1964) Untersuchungen über den antikonvulsiven Wirkungstyp der Kawa-Pyrone Dihydromethysticin und Dihydrokawain mit Hilfe chemisch induzierter Krämpfe. *Archives Internationales des Pharmacodynamie*, 150(1–2), 118–131.

Meyer, H.J. (1966) *Pharmakologie der Kawa-Droge* (Piper methysticum *Forst.)*, Habilitationsschrift, Universität Freiburg, Breisgau.

Meyer, H.J. (1979) Pharmacology of kava. In D.H. Efron, B. Holmstedt and N.S. Kline (eds), *Ethnopharmacologic Search for Psychoactive Drugs*. Raven Press, New York, pp. 131–140.

Meyer, H.J. and Kretzschmar, R. (1966) Kawa-Pyrone eine neuartige Substanzgruppe zentraler Muskelrelaxantien von Typ des Mephenesins. *Klinische Wochenschrift*, 15, 902–903.

Meyer, H.J. and Kretzschmar, R. (1969) Untersuchungen über Beziehunhen zwischen Molekularstruktur und pharmakologischer Wirkung C6-arylsubstituierter 4-Methoxy-alpha-pyrone vom Typ der Kawa-Pyrone. *Arzneimittelforschung*, 19, 617–623.

Meyer, H.J. and May, H.U. (1964) Lokalanaesthetische Eigenschaften natürlicher Kawa-Pyrone. *Klinische Wochenschrift*, 8, 407.

Meyer, H.J., Oberdorff, A. and Seifen, E. (1960) Pharmakologische Untersuchungen über die Wirkstoffe von Kawa-kawa (*Piper methysticum*). *Naunyn Schmiedeberg's Archives of Experimental Pathology and Pharmacology*, 238, 124–125.

Morrison, J. (1935) *The Journals of James Morrison*. Golden Cockerel Press, London. p. 151.

Muir, C., Waterhouse, J., Mack, T., Powell, J. and Whelan, S. (1987) *Cancer Incidents in Five Continents*, International Agency for Research on Cancer, Lyon, pp. 75–82.

Münte, T.F., Heinze, H.J., Matzke, M. and Steitz, J. (1993) Effects of oxazepam and an extract of kava rhizomes (*Piper methysticum*) on event-related potentials in a word recognition task. *Neuropsychobiology*, 27, 46–53.

Neuronika® (1989) *D,L-Kavain, Wissenschaftliche Informationsbroschüre, Klinge Pharma*, Munich, Germany.

Norton, S.A. and Ruze, P. (1994) Kava dermopathy. *Journal of the American Academy of Dermatology*, 31, 89–97.

Olsen, R.W. and Tobin, A.J. (1990) Molecular biology of GABA_A receptors. *FASEB. Journal*, 4, 1812–1823.

Paksoy, N., Montevalli, B. and McCarthy, S.W. (1990) Cancer occurrence in Vanuatu. *Tropical and Geographical Medicine*, 42, 157–161.

Paksoy, N., Bouchardy, C. and Parkin, D. (1991) Cancer incidence in Western Samoa. *International Journal of Epidemiology*, 20, 634–641.

Palmer, M., O'Donnell, J. and Ye, M. (1999) Kava's methysticin: Protection from strychnine and veratridine. *Journal of Toxicology and Clinical Toxicology*, 37(5), 609.

Pfeiffer, C.C., Murphree, H.B. and Goldstein, L. (1979) Effect of kava in normal subjects and patients. In D.H. Efron, B. Holmstedt and N.S. Kline (eds), *Ethnopharmacologic Search for Psychoactive Drugs*, Raven Press, New York, pp. 155–161.

Prescott, J., Jamieson, D., Emdur, N. and Duffield, P. (1993) Acute effects of kava on measures on measures of cognitive performance, physiological function and mood. *Drug and Alcohol Review*, 12, 49–58.

Rasmussen, A.K., Scheline, R.R. and Solheim, E. (1979) Metabolism of some kava pyrones in the rat. *Xenobiotica*, 9(1), 1–16.

Rataud, J., Debarnot, F., Mary, V., Pratt, J. and Stutzman, J.M. (1994) Comparative study of voltage-sensitive sodium channel blockers in focal ischaemia and electric convulsions in rodents. *Neuroscience Letters*, 172, 19–23.

Rex, A., Morgenstern, E. and Fink, H. (2002) Anxiolytic-like effects of kava-kava in the elevated plus maze test – a comparison with diazepam. *Progress in Neuro-Psychopharmacology & Biological Psychiatry*, 26, 855–860.

Russell, P.N., Bakker, D. and Singh, N.N. (1987) The effects of kava on alerting and speed of access of information from long-term memory. *Bulletin of the Psychonomic Society*, 25, 236–237.

Russmann, S., Lauterburg, B.H. and Helbling, A. (2001) Kava hepatotoxicity. *Annals of Internal Medicine*, 135, 68–69.

Ruze, P. (1990) Kava-induced dermopathy. A niacin deficiency? *Lancet*, 335(8703), 1442–1445.

Sällström Baum, S., Hill, R. and Rommelspacher, H. (1998) Effect of kava extract and individual kavapyrones on neurotransmitter levels in the nucleus accumbens of rats. *Progress in Neuro-Psychopharmacology and Biological Psychiatry*, 22, 1105–1120.

Saletu, B., Grünberger, J., Linzmayer, L. and Anderer, P. (1989) EEG-brain mapping, psychometric and psychophysiological studies on central effects of kavain: A kava plant derivative. *Human Psychopharmacology*, 4, 169–190.

Sapp, D.W., Witte, U., Turner, D.M., Longoni, B., Kokka, N. and Olsen, R.W. (1992) Regional variation in steroid anesthetic modulation of [35S] TBPS binding to gamma-aminobutyric acid-A receptors in rat brain. *Journal of Experimental Pharmacology and Therapeutics*, 262, 801–808.

Sass, M., Schnabel, S. and Kröger, J. (2001) Akutes Leberversgen durch Kava-Kava – eine seltene Indikation zur Lebertransplantation [in German]. *Z Gastroenterol*, 39, 491(P29).

Schelosky, L., Raffauf, C., Jendroska, K., and Poewe, W. (1995) Kava and dopamine antagonism. *Journal of Neurology and Neurosurgical Psychiatry*, 58(5), 639–640.

Schirrmacher, K., Büsselberg, D., Langosch, J.M., Walden, J., Winter, U. and Bingmann, D. (1999) Effects of (±)-kavain on voltage-activated inward currents of dorsal rhizome ganglion cells from neonatal rats. *European Neuropsychopharmacology*, 9, 171–176.

Schmidt, J. (2001) *Analysis of kava side effects. Reports concerning the liver.* Lindenmaier, M. and Brinckmann, J., translators. December 31 2001 (unpublished). Courtesy: American Herbal Products Association, Silver Springs, MD.

Schmitz, D., Zhang, C.L., Chatterjee, S.S. and Heinemann, U. (1995) Effects of methysticin on three different models of seizure like events studied in rat hippocampal and entorhinal cortex slices. *Naunyn Schmiedeberg's Archives of Pharmacology*, 351, 348–355.

Schübel, K. (1924) Zur Chemie und Pharmakologie der Kawa-Kawa (*Piper methysticum*, Rauschpfeffer). *Naunyn Schmiedeberg's Archives of Experimental Pathology and Pharmacology*, 102, 250–282.

Seitz, U., Schüle, A. and Gleitz, J. (1997a) [^{3}H]-Monoamine uptake inhibition properties of kava pyrones. *Planta Medica*, 63, 548–549.

Seitz, U., Amen, A., Pelzer, H., Gleitz, J. and Peters, T. (1997b) Relaxation of evoked contractile activity of isolated guinea-pig ileum by (±)-kavain. *Planta Medica*, 63, 303–306.

Shulgin, A.T. (1973) The narcotic pepper: the chemistry and pharmacology of *Piper methysticum* and related species. *Bulletin of Narcotics*, 25, 59–74.

Siegel, R.H. (1976) Herbal intoxication. *Journal of the American Medical Association*, 236, 473–476.

Siegers, C.P. (1993) Risk assessment of psychotropic phytopharmaceuticals. *Pharmacopsychiatry*, 26, 195.

Singh, K., Singh, K.P. and Seruvatu, I. (1986) *Cancer Occurrence in Developing Countries*, IARC Scientific Publication No. 75, International Agency for Research on Cancer, Lyon, pp. 315–321.

Singh, Y.N. (1983) Effects of kava on neuromuscular transmission and muscle contractility. *Journal of Ethnopharmacology*, 7, 267–276.

Singh, Y.N. (1992) Kava: an overview. *Journal of Ethnopharmacology*, 37, 13–45.

Smith, K.K., Dharmaratne, H.R., Feltenstein, M.W., Broom, S.L., Roach, J.T., Nanayakkara, N.P., *et al.* (2001) Anxiolytic effects of kava extract and kavalactones in the chick social separation-stress paradigm. *Psychopharmacology*, 155, 86–90.

Steiner, G.G. (2000) The correlation between cancer incidence and kava consumption. *Hawaii Medical Journal*, 59, 420–422.

Steinmetz, E.F. (1960) *Piper methysticum*. Published by the author, Amsterdam.

Stoller, R. (2000) Leberschädigungen unter Kava-Extrakten. *Schweizerische Ärztezeitung*, 81, 1335–1336.

Strahl, S., Ehret, V., Dahm, H.H. and Maier, K.P. (1998) Necrotizing hepatitis after taking herbal medication. *Deutsche Medizinische Wochenshrift*, 123, 1410–1414.

Süss, R. and Lehmann, P. (1996) Hematogenous allergic contact dermatitis from kava, an herbal product. *Hautarzt*, 47, 459–461.

Swensen, J. (1996) Man convicted of driving under influence of kava. *Deseret Times*, Salt Lake City, Utah, August 5, p. 9.

Thevenot, H., Germain, R. and Chaubet, M. (1986) *Cancer Occurrences in Developing Countries*, International Agency for Research on Cancer, Lyon, pp. 323–329.

Thomson, B.H. (1908) *The Fijians: A Study of the Decay of Custom*, Heinemann, London, pp. 341–351.

Titcomb, M. (1948) Kava in Hawaii. *Journal of the Polynesian Society*, 57, 105–171.

Uebelhack, R., Franke, L. and Schewe. H.J. (1998) Inhibition of platelet MAO–B by kava pyrone-enriched extract from *Piper methysticum* Forster (kava–kava). *Pharmacopsychiatry*, 31, 187–192.

Van Veen, A.G. (1938) Over de vedwelmende stof uit de kawa-kawa of wati-plant (*Piper methysticum*). *Geneeskund Tijdschrift voor Nederlandsch–Indie*, 78, 194–195.

Walden, J., von Wegerer, J., Winter, U., Berger, M. and Grunze, H. (1997) Effects of kawain and dihydromethysticin on field potential changes in the hippocampus. *Progress in Neuro-psychopharmacology and Biology Psychiatry*, 21, 697–706.

Yamasaki, Y., Kogure, K., Hara, H., Ban, H. and Akaike, N. (1991) The possible involvement of tetrodotoxin–sensitive ion channels in ischemic neuronal damage in rat hippocampus. *Neuroscience Letters*, 121, 251–254.

Young, M.C., Fricker, P.A., Thomson, N.J. and Lee, K.A.P. (1999) Sudden death to ischaemic heart disease in young Aboriginal sportsmen in the Northern Territory, 1982–1996. *Medical Journal of Australia*, 170, 425–428.

7 Kava: Clinical Studies and Therapeutic Implications

Nirbhay N. Singh, Subhashni D. Singh and Yadhu N. Singh

Introduction

Kava has had a long history of use in folk medicine by the traditional healers of Oceania. However, it is now popularly known as an elixir that induces relaxation and sociability, and leads one to a sublime state of being. Before the arrival of European explorers, the peoples of Oceania did not have any knowledge of alcoholic beverages and used kava, a nonalcoholic beverage, as their social drink (Singh, 1992). The islanders had discovered that by chewing fresh or dried kava roots that released the active lipid soluble kavalactones, they could access a potent liquid that could be diluted with water to produce a social beverage. As noted by Lebot (1991), " ... when the beverage is not too concentrated, drinkers attain a state of happy unconcern, well-being and contentment. They feel relaxed and free of any physical or psychological excitement ... the beverage soothes temperaments and drinkers never become angry, unpleasant, noisy or quarrelsome." Early missionaries to the islands prohibited the inhabitants from drinking kava and the practice almost disappeared in some islands, such as Tahiti and Hawaii. However, it remained a social and ceremonial beverage in other islands and has recently emerged as a herbal preparation in many western countries.

Historical uses

Historically, kava has been widely used to treat numerous ailments, diseases, and disorders (Titcomb, 1948; Zepernick, 1972; Singh, 1992; Lebot *et al.*, 1997). Although the beverage was the most commonly used preparation of kava for medicinal purposes, it was also used in other forms to induce healing. For example, a poultice made from kava root pulp was used to treat skin diseases and to prevent suppuration. The leaves were also used to induce abortion, and the roots were eaten to treat headaches. In some places, heated kava leaves were placed on the head to relieve headaches, while the juice from the leaves was used to treat cuts, and in massage for general lethargy and weakness. Drinks made from macerated kava stump were given to alleviate urinary and vaginal problems, fever and chills, rheumatism, obesity, stomach upsets, and asthma. Drinks made from masticated kava were used to treat migraine, pulmonary disorders, and sleeping problems, as well as to prevent infection. In effect, kava was used in different preparations, alone and together with other plants, for a broad range of physical, medical, and emotional disorders (Singh, 1992).

Current clinical uses

In terms of its clinical usage, kava has been evaluated primarily for its ability to reduce anxiety and secondarily for coping with stress and depression (Singh and Singh, 2002). *Anxiety* is a very diffuse mental condition when one has the unpleasant feeling of apprehension but does not know its source. It manifests in a variety of ways including pounding heart, tightness in the chest, tremors, sweating, sleeplessness, and an uncomfortable feeling in the stomach. Low levels of anxiety are common in daily life and most of us cope with it fairly well. When anxiety reaches levels with which we are unable to cope and are constantly on edge, it may be that we have developed an anxiety disorder that requires mental health intervention. Anxiety disorders are probably the most common of the psychiatric disorders, with lifetime prevalence in the range of 15–25%.

Until recently, the benzodiazepines were accepted as the treatment of choice for anxiety disorders. However, benzodiazepines have the potential for abuse, tolerance, dependence, and withdrawal reactions following prolonged use, and rebound after discontinuation. Also, they can increase the intoxicating potency of alcohol. Their common side-effects include sedation, impaired cognition, and motor incoordination (Werry, 1998). Further, benzodiazepines may have behavioral side-effects, including irritability, depression, hyperactivity, aggression, and disinhibition (Van Der Bijl and Roelofse, 1991; Bond, 1998). Thus, there has been a move away from the use of benzodiazepines to other psychotropic drugs, including complementary and alternative medicine approaches to control anxiety. One of the approaches has been the use of kava for both elevated anxiety in daily life and for anxiety disorders as diagnosed according to the DSM-IV criteria (American Psychiatric Association, 1994).

Anxiety is associated with both acute (e.g., job interview) and chronic stressors (e.g., physical illness, sexual or physical abuse) in daily life. While most of us experience many environmental and psychosocial stressors in our life, most do not produce anxiety disorders unless we have some vulnerability or disturbance predating specific stressors (Goodyer, 1990). *Stress* in our daily life increases because of specific events related to our personal life or work environment. When this kind of stress reduces or threatens to reduce our quality of life, we seek help. In addition or as an alternative to medication, we may engage in vigorous physical exercise, yoga, or meditation to reduce stress. Recently, it has been suggested that kava might be helpful in reducing daily stress.

Depression has also been targeted for treatment with kava, as it is a mood disorder that is related to anxiety disorders and psychosocial stress. It has been suggested that kava elevates mood without affecting cognition. Several studies will be discussed that evaluate the effects of kava on both anxiety and depression. This is to be expected because the signs and symptoms of anxiety and depression overlap to a substantial degree: restlessness/mental tension, fatigue, poor concentration, irritability, sleep disturbance, and significant impairment in social and occupational functioning. Kava has also been used for other clinical purposes, for instance as a sleep aid and in the treatment of seizure disorders. Whether we continue to investigate the efficacy of kava for these and other clinical interventions will depend to a large degree not only on its efficacy but also on its unintended side-effects. In this chapter, we review the studies that have investigated the clinical and adverse side-effects of kava.

Clinical Studies

There has been a relatively small number of clinical trials with kava, a majority of them conducted in Germany. Although kava is a herbal anxiolytic drink that is prepared in the South Seas as a water extract, most of the trials have been performed on commercially produced preparations that contain kavalactones extracted using organic solvents, such as ethanol and acetone. The kavalactone content of these formulations usually is between 30 and 70%. In addition, a number of studies have used individual synthetic preparations [e.g., (±)-kavain] rather than kava extracts which contain a mixture of at least six major active kavalactones. Thus, comparisons across studies in terms of clinical efficacy and adverse side-effects should not be made across studies unless they have used similar, standardized kava preparations.

Anxiety

There are three groups of studies on the effects of kava in reducing anxiety: (a) those that included subjects with a diagnosable anxiety disorder or with anxiety symptomatology; (b) those that included individuals with anxiety associated with menopause; and (c) those that included individuals with anxiety due to a medical condition. Further, we can differentiate studies in terms of the type of kava preparation used, that is, those containing kava extracts or synthetic kavalactones.

Anxiety disorders and anxiety symptomatology

A number of studies with subjects that met DSM-IV criteria for anxiety disorders have been reported in the literature. The first involved a 24-week, 10-center, randomized double blind placebo-controlled study of the effects of the kava extract, WS 1490 (Willmar Schwabe, Germany), on non-psychotic anxiety in 101 outpatients (Volz, 1996; Volz and Kieser, 1997). A one-week placebo washout period was included prior to the study, as well as a one-week placebo washout following the 24-week trial. Assessments undertaken at the beginning of the placebo washout period, and at weeks 0, 12, and 24 included: Hamilton Anxiety Scale (HAMA; Hamilton, 1959), a self-report symptom inventory (SCL-90-R; Derogatis, 1994), Clinical Global Impression (CGI; NIMH, 1970), Adjective Mood Scale (BF-S; von Zerssen, 1986), and adverse events (AE) rating on an open non-leading questionnaire. Additional HAMA and AE ratings were undertaken at weeks 4, 8, 16, and 20. Further, another set of assessments were performed after the final one-week placebo washout that followed the 24-week trial.

The total scores on the HAMA scale, the main efficacy variable, decreased for both groups across the 24-week trial. However, the WS 1490 group showed a greater decrease in the HAMA scores than the placebo group at each monitoring, with the difference increasing as the trial progressed. There was a statistically significant difference between the WS 1490 and placebo groups on the HAMA and the HAMA subscale scores beginning at week 8. On the CGI, there was a statistically significant difference between the two groups in terms of the number of outpatients who improved in their psychopathological state. The superiority of the WS 1490 group on the SCL-90-R ratings was evident starting at 12 weeks of treatment and continuing to the end of the trial.

Five patients in the WS 1490 group reported having six AEs, but four of the six AEs were unrelated to the WS 1490; the other two were stomach upsets that could have been due to the kava extract or some other factor. Nine patients in the placebo group reported having 15 AEs. Three patients dropped out of WS 1490 group, two because they said their condition had improved and the other for noncompliance. Six patients dropped out of the placebo group. This long-term placebo-controlled trial of a kava extract showed that it was more effective than placebo in both the short- and long-term treatments of nonpsychotic anxiety and that it was a safe product, having few adverse events.

In another study, Malsch and Kieser (2001) investigated the anxiolytic effects of WS 1490 compared to placebo in patients previously treated with a benzodiazepine. They evaluated the potential of the kava preparation as a replacement for the benzodiazepine, as well as the ability of the kava preparation to reduce benzodiazepine withdrawal symptoms. This was a five-week randomized, double blind placebo-controlled study in outpatients with non-psychotic anxiety (e.g., generalized anxiety disorder, social phobia, and simple phobia). Forty patients were included, and all had been on benzodiazepines (i.e., lorazepam, bromazepam, oxazepam, or alprazolam) for a mean duration of 20 months prior to entering the study. Of the 40 patients, 25 were males, and the mean age of the total sample was 40 years (range 21–75 years).

During the first week of the trial, the treatment group received WS 1490, beginning at a dose of 50 mg/day and increasing to 300 mg/day by the end of the week. The benzodiazepines previously prescribed to both the kava and placebo groups were gradually tapered during weeks 1 and 2. The kava group received WS 1490 at 300 mg/day for the following three weeks and the placebo group received placebo alone. This was followed by a three-week follow-up phase during which the patients who had showed no or minimal improvement during the trial received anxiolytic treatment according to the clinical judgment of the investigating physician. The primary outcome measures of improvement included the total HAMA score and ratings on a subjective well-being scale. CGI was a secondary measure of overall outcome. Adverse events were also recorded.

The WS 1490 preparation was found to be statistically superior to placebo in reducing anxiety in the absence of adjunctive benzodiazepines. Enhanced patient functioning was evident within the first week of kava therapy, and improvements continued during the course of the five-week trial. There were some data to support the contention that the kava preparation was superior to the effects of benzodiazepines and that kava mitigated the withdrawal effects of the benzodiazepines. The pattern of responses on the primary and secondary outcomes measures was similar for both groups. Adverse events were reported by five patients in the kava group and ten patients in the placebo group. In all cases, the adverse events were related to the withdrawal of the benzodiazepines, and no adverse events were attributable to the kava. During the follow-up phase, four patients in the kava group and 11 in the placebo group who had not shown clinically significant improvements in their symptoms received standard anxiolytic treatment for their conditions.

More recently, Connor and Davidson (2002) evaluated the efficacy and safety of kava in treating generalized anxiety disorder (GAD). Thirty-seven adults who met the DSM-IV criteria for GAD were randomly assigned to four weeks of double blind treatment with kava or a matching placebo. Treatment was initiated at 70 mg kavalactones (kl) twice a day for one week (140 mg kl/day) and increased to 140 mg kl twice a day (280 mg kl/day) for the next three weeks. Weekly efficacy assessments using the HAMA, Self Assessment of Resilience and Anxiety (SARA; Barnett *et al.*, 2001) and

Hospital Anxiety and Depression Scale (HADS; Zigmond and Snaith, 1983) and safety, monitored by evaluation of vital signs, laboratory and EKG assessments pre- and post-treatment, medications side-effects, and withdrawal symptoms, were conducted. Improvement was observed with both treatments, but no differences were found in the principal analysis. Post-hoc analyses revealed significant differences based on the severity of baseline anxiety, whereby kava was superior on the SARA in low anxiety and placebo was superior on the HADS and SARA in high anxiety. The treatments were well tolerated and there was no evidence of withdrawal or sexual side-effects. The authors concluded that although kava was not superior to placebo in this trial, it would be premature to rule it out as a possible treatment for GAD.

Nine other studies involved subjects with anxiety symptomatology but not clinically diagnosed as an anxiety disorder. The first three of these used (±)-kavain, a synthetic kavalactone, and the remaining six studies used different kava preparations. With the exception of two studies (Scherer, 1998; Boerner, 2001), all used a double blind, placebo-controlled experimental design.

Möller and Heuberger (1989) assessed the effects of (±)-kavain in a double blind, placebo-controlled study on 40 outpatients with symptoms of anxiety. All patients were described as having anxiety-related neurotic or psychosomatic disturbances. Baseline and end-point measures included a standardized self-rating scale for symptomatology and physicians' clinical global ratings. Following a one-week washout period, the patients were given either an oral administration of $3 \times 200\,mg$ (±)-kavain/day or placebo for two weeks. The results showed a statistically significant reduction in self-reported symptoms of anxiety in the kavain group as compared to the placebo group. In the physicians' ratings, 80% of the kavain group and 40% of the placebo group showed either good or very good improvement in anxiety symptoms at the end of the two-week study period. The authors concluded that their study provided empirical and clinical evidence of the anxiolytic properties of kavain.

Lehmann and coworkers (1989) conducted a three-center, double blind placebo-controlled trial of (±)-kavain (Neuronika®)[1]. Of the 56 patients included in the study, four dropped out within the first two weeks of treatment due to reasons unrelated to the study. Of the 52 remaining patients, 21 had a panic syndrome, 17 had generalized anxiety syndrome, 10 disturbance of adaptability, and 4 phobic disturbances. No details were provided in terms of gender. The average age of the total sample was about 40 years. None of the patients were on psychotropic medication for any of the conditions.

The 52 patients were assigned to two groups (active and placebo) counterbalanced for age, duration of illness, clinical status on the Minnesota Multiphasic Personality Inventory (MMPI; Greene, 1980), and scores on the HAMA scale. The active treatment group daily received $2 \times 200\,mg$ kavain or placebo for a period of 28 days. In addition to the baseline HAMA, outcomes were assessed on days 14 and 28 on HAMA, Adjective Checklist, physicians' global impressions, and patient reports of side-effects.

It was found that the kavain-treated group had lower scores (i.e., showing clinical improvement) on the HAMA when compared to the placebo group at both the 14-day and 28-day assessments. Further, there was a time-course effect, with a 35% reduction at the first assessment and about 50% reduction by the end of the trial. Exploratory analysis of the HAMA subscales showed that major reductions were evident on the

---

1 The use of trade names is for product identification purposes only.

'psychic anxiety' and 'somatic anxiety' subscales. At the end of the trial, there was only about 13% reduction in the HAMA score for the placebo group. On the physicians' global ratings, 21 of 26 patients showed improvement or marked improvement for the kavain group, compared to 7 of 26 for the placebo group. Patients self-rating on the Adjective Checklist showed that kavain resulted in enhanced vitality-related activities and marked reductions in anxiety/depression. Further, there were no clinically significant adverse effects for both groups. The active group also reported that kavain-induced sound sleep and physical relaxation.

Lindenberg and Pitule-Schödel (1990) reported a double blind, placebo-controlled study comparing the effects of (±)-kavain (Neuronika®) and oxazepam on anxiety. The kava dose was 3×200 mg/day compared to 20 mg/day of oxazepam for a period of 28 days. Of the 40 patients enrolled, 38 completed the study. All 38 had a diagnosis of anxiety associated with neurotic or psychosomatic disturbances. Outcome was measured using the Anxiety Status Inventory and the Zung Self-Rating Anxiety Scale (Zung, 1965). In the dosages used, it was evident that the kava preparation and oxazepam were equally effective in terms of their ability to control anxiety in these patients, without having any clinically significant adverse reactions.

In a six-week trial, the effects of the kava extract WS 1490 (300 mg/day; equivalent to 210 mg kavalactones/day), oxazepam (15 mg/day), and bromazepam (9 mg/day) on non-psychotic anxiety were compared in 172 outpatients (Woelk *et al.*, 1993). A number of variables were monitored, including HAMA and CGI, at baseline and weeks 1, 3, and 6 of the trial. The total scores on the HAMA were not significantly different across the three active drugs, suggesting that the kava preparation was as effective as the benzodiazepines.

Lehmann *et al.* (1996; also published as Kinzler *et al.*, 1991) studied the clinical efficacy and tolerance of WS 1490 in outpatients with anxiety, tension, and excitedness. This was a randomized, double blind, placebo-controlled study. Two groups of 29 patients each received 3×100 mg of WS 1490 or placebo daily for four weeks. The patients were included if they had a baseline total score above 18 on the HAMA Scale, aged between 18 and 60 years, and not on any psychotropic medications during this study. All 58 subjects (43 females) were assessed at baseline and after 7, 14, and 28 days on the trial. The outcomes variables included the total HAMA score, the two HAMA subscales (mental anxiety and somatic anxiety), scores on the Adjectives Checklist, CGI Scale, and the Fischer's Somatic or Adverse Experiences Checklist. The kava extract produced a statistically significant reduction in the total HAMA score at each of the three assessment points. Reduced anxiety was evident by the end of the first week of the trial. HAMA scores for the placebo group remained practically unchanged. Similar results were observed for the two HAMA subscales. Furthermore, self-assessed anxiety/ depression on the Adjectives Checklist and severity of anxiety on the CGI scores also showed statistically significant decreases for only the WS 1490 group.

No significant adverse events were reported during the course of the trial. Six patients (four from WS 1490 and two from placebo) dropped out of the trial but not because of adverse effects of the WS 1490. Overall, the authors concluded that kava extract WS 1490 was effective in reducing anxiety in a sample of outpatients by statistically and clinically significant levels, without any significant adverse effects. Further, the efficacy was evident within a week of initiating the trial.

Singh and coworkers (1998) reported a randomized, double blind placebo-controlled, fixed-dose study of kava (Kavatrol®) within a parallel groups design. Sixty individuals (32 females; mean age = 37 years) from the general population, who had elevated levels of daily stress and anxiety, participated in a four-week trial. Each subject received 2×120 mg kavalactones or placebo capsules daily. Baseline data collected included the SCL-90 score; medical history, including previous treatments for non-clinical anxiety and daily stress; socio-demographic information; Daily Stress Inventory (DSI); State-Trait Anxiety Inventory (STAI); Untoward Effects Checklist; and vital signs (blood pressure, heart rate, and respiratory rate). Outcome data on the DSI and STAI were collected once each week, on the same day, for four weeks. Adverse effects data were collected daily on the Untoward Effects Checklist. The data obtained indicated that daily stress due to interpersonal problems, personal competency, cognitive stressors, environmental hassles, and varied stressors as measured on the DSI was significantly reduced for the kava group. State anxiety was also significantly reduced for the subjects receiving kava. However, there was no significant difference in trait anxiety, a fairly fixed attribute in humans, for the subjects in both the kava and placebo groups. When compared to baseline levels, none of the subjects experienced a worsening in any of the 27 side-effects parameters as a consequence of taking kava or placebo capsules.

The authors concluded that kava reduced daily stress and nonclinical levels of anxiety in adults when compared to baseline and placebo conditions. This was the first study to show that kava reduces the stress that is associated with the daily hassles of life. In addition, it was found that overall stress decreased as a function of the time that a person was on kava.

Scherer (1998) reported a seven-center, open, observational study of a kava preparation, Kavasedon®. The study included 52 outpatients (37 females) with a diagnosis of nonpsychotic anxiety, including agoraphobia, other specific phobias, generalized anxiety disorder, and adjustment disorder with anxiety. Half of the patients also had a secondary diagnosis of depression. The 25 patients who were already being treated with various psychotropic drugs for their anxiety disorders discontinued them when the kava treatment was initiated. Of the total sample, 27 had various other medical conditions (e.g., diseases or disorders of the circulatory system, nervous system, musculoskeletal system, connective tissue, endocrine, and skin), 24 of whom received medication for the medical condition during the kava trial.

All 52 patients received a unit dosage of 100 mg/day of kava extract. The treatment duration varied across subjects, with a mean of about 51 days across the total sample. The patients rated their treatment outcome on the Global Improvement Scale using a five-point rating system. Physicians rated the three target symptoms (anxiety, tension, and restlessness) on a four-point scale: not present, mild, moderate, and severe. In addition, information on adverse events was obtained through a questionnaire.

The results showed that nine patients (17%) rated their treatment as "very good" on the Global Improvement Scale, 33 as "good," 7 as "fair," and 3 as "poor." The physicians" ratings showed marked reductions in the levels of the target symptoms, with 20 patients (39%) reporting no anxiety, 15 (29%) with no tension, and 18 (35%) with no restlessness by the end of the trial. According to the author, the study confirmed the effectiveness of kava in reducing or controlling anxiety under everyday conditions. What is particularly notable is the fact that kava was effective in many patients who were previously on psychotropic medication for the same problem. The data are impressive although they are derived from an uncontrolled trial and volunteer subjects with mixed diagnoses of anxiety and concomitant medical conditions. However, the study was designed to approximate the conditions under which many people would use over-the-counter alternative therapies in their lives, and it showed positive results for kava.

In a Brazilian multicenter study, the efficacy and tolerability of the kava extract, WS 1490, was evaluated in 766 adults (574 females), whose average age was 42.8 years (Toniolo Neto, 1999). All were diagnosed as suffering from some form of anxiety. They were given a dose of 3×100 mg/day of WS 1490 for four weeks. At the end of the trial, there was a 70% reduction in HAMA scores when compared to baseline, and tolerability was rated from 'good' to 'very good' in about 96% of the subjects. The author concluded that WS 1490 was effective in treating anxiety, tension, insomnia, and muscular symptoms (e.g., pain and fatigue).

Boerner (2001) reported the case of a 37-year old woman who suffered from generalized anxiety disorder, simple phobia (fear of flying), and a specific social phobia (public speaking). She did not have panic attacks, agoraphobia, or depressive disorder. A course of psychotherapy had proven unsuccessful and the patient avoided treatment with psychotropic drugs because she feared addiction to benzodiazepines and impaired cognitive functioning. She was treated with the kava preparation LI 150 in a daily dose of 135 mg kavalactones for six months without adjunctive therapies. Subjective improvement in levels of anxiety symptoms and specific phobias were noted at week 1. Improvements continued, and the patient reported reduction of anxiety and phobias by about 75% by the end of four weeks. Reductions were reported on several measures, including CGI, HAMA, Hamilton Depression Scale, Beck Anxiety Inventory, Speilberger Trait Anxiety Inventory, and the Speilberger State Anxiety Inventory. Further reductions were evident at 12 weeks. When assessed at six months following the initiation of the kava therapy, the patient was functioning with close to normal scores on all outcomes measures. She did not report any adverse effects due to the kava preparation.

In a study to evaluate whether kava or valerian could moderate the effects of stress under controlled conditions, 54 subjects (30 females) participated in a standardized color/word mental stress task (Cropley *et al.*, 2002). Following completion of a baseline mental stress session (T1), the participants were randomly assigned to one of three equally sized experimental groups. For the next 7 days, one group received nothing and acted as non-placebo controls, while the remaining two groups received a standard daily dose of either kava (120 mg, LI 150) or valerian (600 mg, LI 156). Seven days later, the participants completed an identical stress testing session (T2).

Blood pressure (BP), heart rate (HR), and subjective ratings of pressure were assessed at rest and during the mental stress task. Differences in BP and HR from resting levels were rated as reactions to the stress task at both time points. At T2, systolic BP responsivity showed a significant decrease in both kava and valerian groups compared to T1, but there was no significant change in diastolic BP. Between T1 and T2, the HR reaction to mental stress declined in the valerian group but not in the kava group. Participants taking kava or valerian reported less pressure during the task at T2 relative to T1. There were no significant differences in BP, HR, or subjective reports of pressure between T1 and T2 in the control group. Behavioral performance on the color/word task did not change among all the groups over the two time points. The data indicate that kava and valerian may be beneficial to health by reducing physiological reactivity during stressful situations.

Anxiety associated with menopause

Three studies investigated the effects of kava extracts on anxiety associated with peri- and post-menopause. Warnecke *et al.* (1990) assessed the effects of kava extract WS 1490 on 40 menopausal women in a double blind, placebo-controlled study. The kava group was given 300 mg (210 mg kavalactones)/day during the four-week trial. When compared to the placebo group, the kava group of women had significant reductions in anxiety. Of these, five reported adverse effects, mainly headaches, tiredness, and a lack of energy.

In a similar study, Warnecke (1991) reported a randomized, double blind placebo-controlled study of WS 1490 with 40 peri- and post-menopausal women between the ages of 45 and 60 years. The women were randomized into two groups, one receiving the kava extract 3×100 mg/day and the other receiving a placebo preparation for a period of eight weeks. The primary outcome variable was the HAMA overall score of anxiety symptomatology. The secondary variables included menopausal symptoms rated on the Kuppermann Index and Schneider scale, and ratings on the Depression Status Inventory (DSI) and the CGI scale. Assessments were taken at baseline and weeks 1, 4, and 8 of the trial. The results showed a statistically significant reduction in the HAMA overall score only in the kava group, indicative of clinically significant improvement in anxiety symptomatology. This improvement was evident from the first week of the study. When compared to the control group, the kava group also showed greater reductions in depressed mood, increased subjective well-being, decreased severity on the CGI, and decreased menopausal symptoms. There were no adverse effects that warranted intervention or withdrawal from the study.

Recently, De Leo *et al*. (2000) investigated the adjunctive effects of a kava extract on anxiety in postmenopausal women. Of the 40 women included in the trial, 22 were in physiological menopause and 18 in surgical menopause. All of them were on hormone replacement therapy (estrogen 50 µg/day with progestin). In the trial, 24 women (13 physiological and 11 surgical menopause) were given adjunctive kava (100 mg/day) and 16 women were given placebo. At three and six months on these two combinations, all women showed a significant decline in their anxiety scores on the HAMA. However, those on adjunctive kava showed a greater reduction in their HAMA anxiety scores when compared to those on hormones alone. De Leo and coworkers suggested that kava may be an effective adjunctive therapy for women in stabilized menopause, particularly those suffering from anxiety because kava assists in the resolution of psychological symptoms without affecting the therapeutic action of estrogen.

Anxiety due to medical conditions

Three studies assessed the effects of kava on anxiety precipitated by a medical condition. Bhate *et al*. (1989) used a kava extract with 59 preoperative patients in a double blind, placebo-controlled study. The patients were given 300 mg of kava (90 mg kavalactones) the night before and 300 mg kava an hour before their operation. Their anxiety, which was rated before and after the operation on a ten-point scale, showed that when compared to the placebo group, the kava group had a significant reduction in the anxiety level. Two of the patients in the kava group reported post-operative hangover, although it was unclear if this was a residual effect of anesthesia or the kava.

Staedt *et al*. (1991) assessed the effects of (±)-kavain on anxiety in 60 patients with tuberculosis or awaiting its diagnosis. The trial was a randomized, double blind placebo-controlled 12-week study. When evaluated on the Hamilton Depression Scale, patients receiving kavain showed statistically significant improvement compared to patients on placebo treatment.

The anxiolytic effects of a kava preparation (Kavasporal Forte®) were examined by Neuhaus *et al.* (2000) in a randomized placebo-controlled trial in 20 patients with acute anxiety. These patients were awaiting the results of a histopathological diagnosis for suspected mammary carcinoma. When compared to placebo, a week's treatment with the kava product significantly reduced their anxiety as well as symptoms of depression. No adverse effects were reported by any of the patients.

In summary, these studies indicate that synthetic kavalactones and kava extract preparations alike are effective in managing anxiety disorders and anxiety symptomatology in a wide array of individuals. Kava was found to be as effective as the benzodiazepines but without their adverse effects. Further, the few adverse effects associated with kava were minor and transient in nature. However, the database on the clinical effects of kava by itself, and in comparison to and together with other psychotropic agents, is currently very small. This is an area ripe for further well-controlled, multi-center studies.

Sleep and insomnia

In a double blind, randomized, placebo-controlled study, the effect of a 150 mg or 300 mg dose of kava extract (Laitan®) was examined on the sleep pattern of 12 healthy volunteers (Emser and Bartylla, 1991). Although both doses were effective, only the higher dose was significantly superior over the placebo in latency, duration, and quality of sleep according to objective measures and subjective reports.

Wheatley (2001) reported an uncontrolled trial of the effects of kava and valerian on sleep in 24 patients suffering from stress-induced insomnia. In Phase I, the 24 patients were treated with a dose of 120 mg kavalactones/day for six weeks. This was followed by a two-week period when they were not on any treatment. Five patients dropped out during this period. In Phase II, the remaining 19 patients were treated with a dose of 600 mg valerian/day for another six weeks. Three areas of stress (social, personal, and life events) and three areas of insomnia (time to fall asleep, hours slept, and waking mood) were assessed. Wheatley found that in the doses tested, both kava and valerian significantly and equally reduced total stress and insomnia. About 58% of the patients reported no side-effects from either compound. For those reporting side-effects, the commonest were vivid dreams with valerian (16%) and dizziness with kava (12%). The finding that kava may be effective in reducing daily stress is in accord with the findings of Singh *et al.* (1998). However, the Wheatley study was an uncontrolled trial and thus the findings need to be replicated in well-controlled comparative trials of kava and valerian.

Seizure management

Pfeiffer and coworkers (1979) investigated the effects of kava in controlling seizures. They found that 6 g/day of a water extract when given to nine selected participants provided good protection against seizures that previously were uncontrolled. A similar degree of control was achieved with 1.0 g/day of an alcohol extract. Kava therapy was discontinued after several weeks due to skin reaction from both the water and alcohol extracts. A further study was undertaken but with synthetically produced (±)-dihydromethysticin. An unreported number of patients with seizure disorder were given doses up to 1.2 g/day of the water extract for four weeks. Apparently grand mal seizures decreased without affecting petit mal seizures. The trial had to be terminated after four weeks because of conjunctival and circumorbital erythema, vomiting, and diarrhea reported by some of the patients. Also, the report was lean with respect to details of the participants, the methodology used, outcome data, and the classification of seizures. Further, no data were presented on the use of any concurrent antiepileptic drugs (AED). Recent studies indicating that kavalactones possess pharmacological mechanisms of action that may produce antiseizure activity are discussed in Chapter 6 and involve possible interaction with $GABA_A$ receptors and Na^+ channel blockade. These findings suggest that there is a theoretical possibility of using kava for seizure management.

Cognitive function

There has been limited and unsystematic assessment of the effects of kava on various cognitive functions. Scholing and Clausen (1997) undertook a double blind, placebo-controlled study of the effects of (±)-kavain (Neuronika®) on 84 participants with vegetative symptoms as measured on Eysenck's MMQ personality inventory. There were two kavain groups and two placebo control groups: 16 subjects (kavain) aged between 20 and 40 years; 16 (placebo) aged between 20 and 40 years; 26 (kavain) aged between 30 and 55 years; and 26 (placebo) aged between 30 and 55 years. The unit dose was 2×200 mg/day of Neuronika® for the kavain group and simultaneous placebo for the control group, given for a period of three weeks. Repeated measurements were taken on a battery of psychophysiological measures, including memory functions, vigilance, fluency of mental functions, reaction time, and of circulation functions controlled by a 100-watt ergometer. The authors reported that there was a positive increase in all these functions during the three weeks of testing but only in the kavain group. Further, there were no age related effects.

Russell *et al.* (1987) assessed the effects of two doses of a kava drink on alertness (Posner, 1978) and the speed of access of information from long-term memory (Hunt, 1978), using a variant of Posner's letter-match task. In the first study (low dose), 30 g of kava powder was extracted with water and the resulting infusion was made up to 250 ml with water. The participants each drank 50 ml of the infusion 30 minutes prior to testing. For the high dose, a different group consumed 100 ml each of kava of the same strength one hour prior to testing. The control groups consumed the same volume of water. Compared to the control group, both doses of kava drink produced no significant effect on the rise time or magnitude of the alerting function of a warning signal, or on the speed of activation of verbal information in long-term memory.

The acute effects of kava on measures of cognitive performance, physiological functions, and mood were tested in 24 kava-naïve subjects who were randomly assigned either to the kava or control (fruit juice) condition (Prescott *et al.*, 1993). The kava drink was prepared by infusing 200 g of powdered kava roots in 1000 ml of water for about 10 minutes. The kava group of 12 subjects shared 500 ml of this liquid mixed with 500 ml of fruit juice and the control group of 12 shared 1000 ml of fruit juice alone. The addition of fruit juice to kava is not customary in the South Pacific and how it interacts with the kava drink is unknown. Subjects receiving kava reported feeling of intoxication approximately an hour after kava ingestion. Apart from increased body sway in the kava subjects, there were no significant differences between the kava and control groups in heart rate, respiration rate, blood pressure, or on any of the five measures included in the cognitive performance test battery.

The comparative effects of oxazepam and a kava extract on event-related brain potentials (ERPs) in a word recognition task and behavioral measures of cognitive functioning were evaluated by Münte and coworkers (1993). Research has shown that the ERP provides a very sensitive method for assessing the effects of psychotropic drugs (Callaway, 1983). ERPs, which are scalp-recorded electrical potentials generated by neural activity associated with specific sensory, cognitive, and motor processes, "reflect the continuum of processes between stimulus and response, thereby providing information about their time course, neuronal strength and cerebral localization" (Münte *et al.*, 1993).

This was a double blind, crossover design study in which the 12 subjects served as their own controls. The experimental phases were separated by 12 days to allow for drug washout between conditions. There were three phases: placebo; kava extract (WS 1490) 3×200 mg/day for five days; and oxazepam 1×15 mg on the day before testing. In the word recognition task, the results showed that, when compared to the placebo phase, there was a marked slowing of reaction time and a reduction in the number of correct responses in the oxazepam phase, and a nonsignificant increase in the number of correct responses in the kava phase. These data suggest that kava enhance performance memory while oxazepam impairs it in a word recognition paradigm. In related research, Heinze *et al.* (1994), using the same methodology and procedures as in the Münte *et al.* (1993) study, investigated the pharmacopsychological effects of WS 1490, oxazepam, and placebo in a parallel visual search paradigm. The oxazepam caused deficits in automatic feature registration, allocation of attention, and the availability of processing capacity, while kava had a positive effect on the allocation of attention and processing capacity.

Gessner and Cnota (1994) reported a double blind, crossover study of the effects of a standardized kava extract (Antares®120, containing 120 mg kavalactones), diazepam, and placebo on EEG and psychophysiological tests. The experimental phases were separated by seven days to allow for drug washout between crossovers. There were three experimental conditions: Antares® 1×120 mg/day; diazepam 1×10 mg/day; and placebo one tablet. Twelve healthy volunteers completed all conditions, with the subjects serving as their own controls. Testing was scheduled immediately before, then 2 hours, and 6 hours after ingestion of the drugs or placebo. Both kava and diazepam increased the relative intensities of the slow waves but decreased those for alpha waves of the EEG. However, unlike for diazepam, benzodiazepine-specific increase of beta-activity was not recorded with the kava product. In the psychophysiological tests, the critical flicker frequency was reduced more by the two drugs than by the placebo. The subjects also showed performance improvements on a simple reaction time test and complex multiple choice reaction time tests only during the kava condition. This study suggested that kava decreases reaction time under controlled conditions.

That kava appears to have a variable effect on human cognition is not altogether surprising if we examine the historical and ethnographic literature. For instance, Hocart (1929) noted that, "(Kava) gives a pleasant, warm and cheerful, but lazy feeling, sociable though not hilarious or loquacious; the reason is not obscured," and Lemert (1967) observed that, "The head is affected pleasantly... you cannot hate with kava in you. Kava quiets the mind; the world gains no new color or rosy tint; it fits in its place and in one easily understandable whole." Sometimes the effects on other parts of the body may be quite severe, without affecting cognitive function, as found by Morrison (1935), who visited Tahiti between 1788 and 1791, "(Kava) almost immediately deprives them of the use of their limbs and speech, but does not touch the mental faculty and they appear in a thoughtful mood...." However, in other Pacific countries fairly extreme effects of kava on both the mind and the body have been described, for instance, "Under the unrestrained influence of their intoxicating draught, in their appearance and actions, they resembled demons more than human beings" (Ellis, 1828).

Speculation that these effects may, in part, be due to the particular variety or cultivar that was utilized in preparing the kava drink has been given credence by recent studies. In an investigation on the chemotypic diversity of kava in the different island groups of the Pacific, Lebot and Lévesque (1989, 1996) found that there was considerable variation in the total kavalactone content between cultivars and that chemical composition and total kavalactone content were controlled by the genotype rather than external environmental factors. It has also been shown that the chemotypes that produce the most palatable beverage and favorable psychoactive effects contain high proportions of kavain and methysticin, while those chemotypes that cause undesirable or adverse physiological outcomes possess high proportions of dihydrokavain and dihydromethysticin (Chapter 4, this volume; Lebot and Lévesque, 1989). As a significant consequence of the chemotypic variations among the cultivars, the islanders generally select for planting only those cultivars that provide the most palatable beverage and reject the others.

In summary, kava appears to have few adverse effects on human functioning. However, there is reason to be cautious in its use because we have limited data from well-controlled experimental studies and clinical trials. Further, there is a paucity of studies on the long-term effects of kava on human cognitive functioning.

Adverse Effects

Tolerability surveillance

Two major postmarketing surveillance studies have been conducted to evaluate the tolerability of two commercial kava preparations. The first study monitored 4049 adults taking daily 150 mg of kava extract WS 1490 (Laitan®), containing 105 mg of kavalactones, for six weeks (Siegers *et al.*, 1992). Based on the assessment of the attending physician, the tolerability of kava was judged to be "good" or "very good" in 96% of the patients. A total of 61(1.5%) adverse events were reported. These were mainly allergic reactions or gastrointestinal complaints and were mild and readily reversible. A causal relationship was rated as probable by the attending physician in about 50% of the cases. For the remainder, causality was considered improbable or was not evaluated. No herb–drug interactions were reported by any of the subjects taking concomitant medications.

In the other study, 3029 adults took one or two tablets daily of a kava extract (Antares® 120) standardized to 120 mg kavalactones (Hoffmann and Winter, 1996). Tolerability was rated by the attending physician as "good" or "very good" in 93% of the subjects. Adverse events were reported in 69 (2.3%) subjects, 37 (1.2%) of whom withdrew from the study. The most common reports were of allergic reactions, gastrointestinal complaints, and central nervous system symptoms such as headache or dizziness. None of the symptoms were considered serious and disappeared when kava was discontinued.

Physical and cutaneous effects

Acute effects of kava drink, as prepared in the South Pacific countries, may lead to such reversible conditions as anesthesia of the mouth (especially the tongue and oral mucosa), sedation, euphoria, muscle weakness, and ataxia (Frater, 1958; Gajdusek, 1979; Meyer, 1979; Cawte, 1985). However, most of the data on physical effects of the kava drink are anecdotal and not derived from controlled studies. Nevertheless, the consistency of the reports from many sources indicates that these effects are reproducible to a great extent and probably are largely authentic.

Mathews *et al.* (1988) conducted a comparative study of 39 kava users and 34 non-users in an Aboriginal community in northern Australia to assess the long-term effects of kava usage. They divided the kava drinkers into three groups: occasional drinkers (100 g/week); heavy drinkers (310 g/week); and very heavy drinkers (440 g/week). Self reported measures of other substance abuse (e.g., alcohol, cigarettes, petrol-sniffing) were also obtained. The findings indicated that drinking more than socially accepted quantities of kava might lead to "malnutrition and weight loss, liver and renal dysfunction, a rash, red eyes, shortness of breath and possibly incoordination and pulmonary hypertension, as well as abnormalities in red cells, lymphocytes and platelets." Although the authors claimed a causal relationship between kava and these physical outcomes, this study basically was a survey and, at best, only strong correlations can be assumed. Prospective controlled studies are needed to assess causal relationships between the consumption of the kava drink and physical symptoms. Further, the actual amounts of kava consumed by the participants included in the survey were many times higher, in some cases greater than 50 times, than those socially acceptable.

That excessive kava drinking may result in skin rash – a reversible ichthyosiform eruption that has been termed kava dermopathy – is unquestioned as it has been reported for several centuries (Ruze, 1990; Singh, 1992; Norton and Ruze, 1994). The rash has been described as "a state of scaly exfoliation giving the skin a shriveled appearance" (Lewin, 1886). With heavy drinking, the rash may result in dry itchy patches that may later develop skin lesions – called *kani kani* in Fiji (Frater, 1958). As the South Pacific islanders knew from experience, *kani kani* can be reversed by abstaining from kava drinks until the skin condition clears up, and then drinking at moderate levels. We still do not know the exact cause of kava dermopathy, and a number of traditional legends have been invoked to account for it (Gifford, 1924; Prescott and McCall, 1988). Hypotheses about its cause include persistent light reaction and pellagra-like dermatitis (Frater, 1958), accumulation of plant flavopigments (Shulgin, 1973), accumulation of kavalactones (Siegel, 1976), chronic allergic dermatitis (Lebot and Cabalion, 1988), and the kava interfering with cholesterol metabolism (Ruze, 1990). However, with one exception (Ruze, 1990), none of these hypotheses has been tested empirically.

In this study, undertaken with regular kava drinkers on the islands of Tonga, Ruze (1990) tested the assumption that the rash resulting from kava consumption may be related to a niacin deficiency. She randomized 29 kava drinkers into two groups, with one group ($n = 15$) receiving 100 mg niacin (nicotinamide) daily for three weeks and the other group ($n = 14$) receiving placebo. Other than the skin rash, which was attributed to excessive kava consumption, the participants had no other medical or physical complaints. However, all reported red, irritated eyes and increased photosensitivity during periods of heavy drinking. Some study participants (five in the active group and four in the placebo group) reported improvements in the condition of their skin rash and others (two in the active group and three in the placebo group) reported worsening. Thus, it was concluded that oral nicotinamide did not improve the skin condition of heavy kava drinkers. From this study, it appears that kava drinkers do not have a niacin deficiency.

Schelosky and coworkers (1995) reported four cases of patients developing clinical signs that could be attributed to central dopaminergic antagonism due to the ingestion of kava. Case 1 presented with "an acute attack of involuntary neck extension with forceful upward deviation of his eyes, which had begun 90 minutes after the intake of the first dose of Laitan® (100 mg kava extract)." This attack subsided spontaneously within 40 minutes. Case 2 experienced "involuntary oral and lingual dyskinesiae, tonic rotation of the head to the right, and painful twisting movements of the trunk" four hours after her first dose of Laitan®. When this did not subside spontaneously, it was treated successfully with 2.5 mg IM of biperiden. Case 3 experienced "forceful involuntary oral and lingual dyskinesiae" on the fourth day of taking Kavasporal Forte® (3×150 mg/day of kava extract). Treatment with 5 mg IM of biperiden produced immediate suppression of the dyskinesia. With Case 4, dyskinesia worsened after 10 days on Kavasporal Forte® (2×100 mg/day) and returned to baseline level when it was discontinued. The authors speculated that the dyskinesia in these cases was probably caused by the dopaminergic receptor antagonistic properties of the kava extracts.

Visual effects

There is scant literature on the visual effects caused by kava. Anecdotal reports have suggested that drinking kava may cause pupil dilation and reduced light reflexes (Frater, 1958) but this was not borne out by another study (Pfeiffer *et al.*, 1979). These authors administered an oral dose of 800 mg of synthetic (±)-methysticin or its ethyl derivative to two groups of six normal subjects, but found no significant changes in their pupil size.

Garner and Klinger (1985) also investigated the effects of a kava drink on visual functions. They prepared a kava drink as customary in the South Pacific, and gave a single subject 2×300 ml drink at 15 minute intervals. They measured vision using a Snellen chart and refractive error with standard clinical techniques. Near point accommodation, stereoacuity, oculomotor balance, and near point convergence were also determined. The subject's pupil diameter was measured from calibrated biomicroscopic photographs taken during the course of the trial. They found reduced near point of accommodation, increased pupil diameter, decreased near point convergence and disturbed oculomotor balance. The authors suggested that these changes may have been caused by the central nervous effects of kava. However, no changes were noted in refractive error, visual acuity or stereoacuity. Given that this was a single experiment, with a single subject, and only acute effects were measured, these data await replication before we can accept them as normative for the effects of kava on visual functions. The clinical significance of the findings needs to be evaluated as they may impact the capability of kava users to function optimally in situations requiring unimpaired vision.

Hepatotoxicity

In the past few years, about 30 cases of possible hepatotoxicity associated with kava use have been reported from Europe, mostly in Germany and Switzerland, with about 10 additional cases from North America (Hagemann, 2001; Waller, 2002), Australia, and New Zealand. The adverse event reports in these cases included cholestatic hepatitis, icterus (jaundice), increased liver enzymes, liver cell impairment, severe hepatitis with confluent necrosis and irreversible liver damage (requiring transplant in four cases in Europe and two in the US) (Hellwig, 2000; Stoller, 2000; Schmidt, 2001; MMWR, 2002). Although much of the clinical data on most of these cases are either incomplete or generally unavailable (Blumenthal, 2002), relatively detailed information has been published for six of them (Strahl *et al.*, 1998; Brauer *et al.*, 2002; Escher *et al.*, 2001; Kraft *et al.*, 2001; Russmann *et al.*, 2001; Sass *et al.*, 2001). These reports and the alarm caused by them in the print and electronic media have prompted a number of countries in 2002 to take regulatory action to suspend or ban the sale of kava products or issue consumer health advisories on their use (Reuters, 2002). At the time of writing, efforts are under way in a number of laboratories to scientifically substantiate these claims, but it will be some time before the controversy is adequately resolved.

These reports of hepatotoxicity are somewhat contradictory to the experience of South Pacific islanders who have safely used kava for many hundreds of years. In these countries only men consume kava, often habitually and in much larger amounts than used in the west, yet their incidence of liver toxicity is low and similar to that of island women who generally do not take kava. Reviews of the reports of liver toxicity note that in many cases other known or suspected hepatotoxic medications had been administered concurrently. In some cases the use of alcohol or microbial infections had not been ruled out (Schmidt, 2001; Blumenthal, 2002; Waller, 2002). Furthermore, the commercial preparations were manufactured using organic solvents that are confirmed hepatotoxins, such as acetone and ethanol, in contrast to the water infusions drunk by the islanders. Further, in most of the approximately 40 cases cited above, the individuals were also taking pharmaceutical drugs simultaneously. Assuming that these agents were responsible for the adverse events and not some other factors, such as other disease state or excessive alcohol use, it is possible that the hepatotoxicity was caused by the conventional drugs, by the kava, by both the drugs and kava, or mainly by the drugs with kava as a cofactor (Denham *et al.*, 2002). Upon analysis of all relevant factors, the number of cases cited by the government authorities that can actually be attributed to kava alone is very low (Schmidt, 2001). Hence, the logical conclusion that can be drawn is that the relative incidence of adverse effects is a fraction of that associated with established anxiolytics, such as benzodiazepines (Schmidt and Nahrstedt, 2002).

A major way in which an interaction between kavalactones and drugs can occur is by an inhibition of cytochrome P450 enzymes by kavalactones. Since these enzymes are responsible for the hepatic metabolism of many drugs, their inhibition would elevate the plasma concentrations of these agents to toxic levels. The pharmacological evidence in support of this conjecture is addressed later in this chapter.

Kava–drug interactions

Herberg (1993) reported a study that assessed the effects on safety of combining kava with ethanol. This was a double blind, placebo-controlled randomized trial of 40 healthy volunteers (ten males and ten females in each group), aged between 18 and 60 years (mean=41 years). The aim of the study was to test the adverse effects on seven safety-related performance variables when adult volunteers combine kava with acute intake of ethanol at a blood alcohol concentration of 0.05%. The battery of performance tests measured vigilance, coordination, reaction time, and concentration. One group received the kava extract WS 1490 alone, and the other group received the kava extract together with ethanol on days 1, 4, and 8. The kava extract was used at a dosage of 3×100 mg/day over eight days. There were no negative performance effects of combining kava with alcohol when compared to kava alone, except that on day 4, the kava alone group performed significantly better than the kava plus alcohol group ($P < 0.05$). This study suggests that kava and low dose alcohol may not negatively affect performance under controlled conditions.

Another double blind, randomized, crossover study examined the effect of combining a kava extract with a benzodiazepine (Herberg, 1996). Eighteen subjects received daily either 800 mg kava (Antares®), or 9 mg bromazepam, or both for 14 days each. Results from a battery of performance tests indicated no significant differences between bromazepam alone and the combination with kava. Performance with kava alone was no different from baseline values. In all, 77 adverse events were reported, of which 22% were related to kava, 36% to bromazepam, and 42% to the combination. Tiredness was the most common complaint, reported by four subjects taking kava, 11 with bromazepam, and 14 with the combination.

The case of a purported interaction between kava and alprazolam that may have caused a semicomatose state in a 54-year-old man was described by Almeida and Grimsley (1996). The man had been taking alprazolam, cimetidine, and terazosin and, for three days prior to his hospitalization, he self-medicated himself with kava as well. When admitted to the hospital, he was in a lethargic and disoriented state. Tests showed that his vital signs and laboratory values were normal, alcohol was negative, and a positive drug screen for benzodiazepines. Few details, such as dosage of any of the medications or kava, were reported. The authors suggested that kavalactones, and the alprazolam had additive effects because both act on the same GABA receptors and, to support their contention, cited a study by Davies *et al.* (1992). In reality, the latter study concluded that "... the pharmacological activity of the active components of kava are not due to a direct interaction of the kavapyrones with benzodiazepine or GABA receptors." However, it has subsequently been shown that kavalactones do indeed interact with $GABA_A$ receptors but in the brain cortex (Boonen and Haberlein, 1998), not the forebrain and cerebellum which were used by the Davies group, this probably being the reason for their negative results.

Foo and Lemon (1997) assessed the acute effects of kava, alone and in combination with alcohol, on subjective measures of impairment and intoxication and on cognitive performance. This was a placebo-controlled study, with ten subjects in each of four conditions: placebo, kava, alcohol, and kava plus alcohol. The placebo was pure fruit juice and fruit juice was added to kava and alcohol as well to maintain double blind conditions. A battery of tests was included to measure outcomes, including subjective measures of impairment and intoxication, and visual-motor and cognitive performance. These measures were performed before (time=0), and 30, 60 and 90 minutes after consumption of the drinks. Each test trial took about 12 minutes. Kava consumption produced no significant effects on perceived or measured competence, while alcohol caused motor and cognitive impairments. However, when kava and alcohol were combined, kava potentiated both the perceived and measured impairment produced by the alcohol alone. This potentiation effect is in accord with the findings of Jamieson and Duffield (1990) on the positive interaction of ethanol and kava resin in mice.

The possibility of an interaction between kavalactones and pharmaceutical drugs has received some attention since the reports of possible kava-induced hepatotoxicity became available. A major way in which such interaction may occur is by an inhibition of cytochrome P450 (CYP 450) enzymes by kavalactones. Since these enzymes are responsible for the hepatic metabolism of a majority of drugs and xenobiotics, their inhibition could elevate the plasma concentrations of these chemicals to levels that are toxic to various tissues and organs, including the liver.

In a study of the actions of the six major kavalactones on cDNA-derived CYP450 enzymes, Zou and coworkers (2002) found that the most potent inhibition of CYP1A2 occurred with desmethoxyyangonin (IC_{50} 1.70 µM); of CYP2C19 with dihydromethysticin (0.43 µM), desmethoxyyangonin (0.51 µM), and methysticin (0.93 µM); and of CYP3A4 with methysticin (1.49 µM) and dihydromethysticin (2.49 µM). Potent inhibitors in this test were considered to be compounds with IC_{50} values ≤10 µM. What is notable in the data is that kavain, the most potent anxiolytic kavalactone, dihydrokavain, and yangonin were largely ineffective in the highest concentrations tested.

The inhibition of CYP450 enzymes by whole kava extract (containing 100 µM total kavalactones) and individual kavalactones was also investigated in human liver microsomes (Mathews *et al.*, 2002). The extract caused significant inhibition of the activities of CYP1A2 (56% inhibition), 2C9 (92%), 2C19 (86%), 2D6 (73%), 3A4 (78%), and 4A9/11 (65%). CYP2A6, 2C8, and 2E1 activities were unaffected. The activities of CYP2C9, 2C19, 2D6, and 3A4 were measured with kavain, desmethoxyyangonin, methysticin, and dihydromethysticin, each at 10 µM. While kavain did not inhibit these enzymes, there was significant inhibition of CYP2C9 by desmethoxyyangonin (42%), methysticin (58%), and dihydromethysticin (69%); of 2C19 by dihydromethysticin (76%); of 2D6 by methysticin (44%); and of 3A4 by desmethoxyyangonin (40%), methysticin (27%), and dihydromethysticin (54%). These data indicate that kava has a high potential for causing drug interactions through inhibition of CYP450 enzymes responsible for the majority of the metabolism of pharmaceutical agents.

Genetic polymorphism of many CYP enzymes, leading to interindividual variation in drug metabolism, may be another factor in the marked discrepancy in hepatotoxic response to kava of Caucasians from Europe and elsewhere, on the one hand, and the Pacific Islanders, on the other. CYP2D6 is one of the most extensively studied genetically polymorphic enzymes. It is thought to cause much of the interindividual variations seen in drug responses, adverse effects, and interactions with drugs (Poolsup *et al.*, 2000). Individuals may be poor (slow), intermediate, extensive (fast), or ultrafast metabolizers. In a Causasian population 7–9% of individuals are homozygous deficient in CYP2D6 and thus are poor metabolizers (Poolsup *et al.*, 2000). On the other hand, the incidence of CYP2D6 deficiency is almost 0% in persons of pure Polynesian descent and 1% in Asian populations (Wanwirolmuk *et al.*, 1998). Since this enzyme is a major metabolizer of kavalactones, it is tempting to assume that the genetic variability between Caucasian kava users and the Pacific Islanders may be a major contributory factor. It may also explain why the descendants of Asian migrants to the Pacific, like the authors' families, have not reported kava hepatotoxicity. However, the genetic polymorphism of CYP2D6 for Melanesians of Fiji, Vanuatu, and other kava consuming nations or that of other CYP enzymes in the Pacific island populations is yet to be determined.

Quality of Research Evidence

Clearly, there is some evidence for the efficacy of kava in treating everyday anxiety and anxiety due to specific conditions. While it has been touted as one of the main herbal alternatives to benzodiazepines in this regard, this view is based on an extrapolation of the current scientific data. Caution is warranted in the general use of kava for anxiety and related disorders of arousal. There are, as yet, many unanswered questions regarding its efficacy, effectiveness, and safety, especially with regard to the recently reported cases of kava associated hepatotoxicity, as well as its comparative effects with respect to western medicine. A number of critical areas of research and research methodology relevant to kava are briefly discussed below.

Clinical outcomes in kava research have generally been measured using rating scales and clinical impressions. Although the Hamilton Anxiety Scale (HAMA) has been the ubiquitous rating scale in most studies, several other measures have also been used. Some of these have been of local origin and their psychometric properties are not readily available in the literature. It is hoped that as progress is made in evaluating different kava extract preparations, a small number of psychometrically robust instruments will emerge as the standard battery of instruments that can be used so that cross-study comparisons can be made. Further, these instruments need to tap symptoms of specific diagnostic disorders rather than just measure ad hoc categories of physical or mental conditions (e.g., tiredness, lethargy).

In many studies, especially the earlier ones, the inclusion and exclusion criteria for study participants were not clearly articulated. Often heterogeneous groups of participants without a clear explication of their mental health status, either in terms of ICD or DSM classification, were included. In some studies, generic conditions (e.g., anxiety, anxious-depression) rather than specific psychiatric diagnoses were used as the basis for including participants in a study. Further, some studies included participants with diagnosable psychiatric conditions while others used participants who had elevated anxiety or depression that affected their quality of life but not enough for them to seek psychiatric consultation. Future studies should include well-defined inclusionary and exclusionary criteria so that study samples can be replicated across investigations for the purposes of comparison.

The better-designed studies included double blind, placebo-control conditions within a parallel research design. However, most studies did not provide any data on how they randomized or counter-balanced their experimental and placebo or control groups. No studies explicated how they were able to match the two groups in terms of the severity or duration of the subjects' anxiety states. Future studies should use a more robust research methodology, such as a double blind, placebo-controlled, cross over design.

A few case studies were also reported in the literature. These are heuristic for future studies, and it is hoped that future reports of single subjects will move beyond case reports to single subject research methodologies that have proven highly beneficial in drug research (Singh and Beale, 1986). In addition, when single subject cases are reported it behooves the researchers to provide as detailed information as possible about the subject, the kava preparation used, its dosage, concurrent medications or over-the-counter drugs used and their dosages. In the absence of such information, these case reports are not very informative and raise more questions than provide answers. For example, the case report by Almeida and Grimsley (1996) lacks vital information on the prescription medication being used by the person before he began using kava. This field needs to develop a standard data set that needs to be reported in each study so that cross-study comparisons can be made.

Finally, the actual kava product used in research studies bears mentioning. Many German studies used synthetic kavalactones [mostly (±)-kavain] and a kava extract (WS 1490). The latter was standardized for research studies, with 100 mg of WS 1490 containing 70 mg of the active kavalactones. Other researchers have used different kava preparations, each with a unique composition. Further, some researchers have used the kava beverage as currently prepared in the islands in their research. Of course, it may be difficult to standardize the kavalactone content in kava drinks because of the variable composition in the different samples, although kava is sold in the western markets mainly in the form of pharmaceutical preparations which can be easily standardized. The use of kava infusions and unstandardized products has led to a situation where presently it is impossible to compare treatment outcomes, as well as adverse effects, across studies. Perhaps, studies should report dosages in terms of the amounts of kavalactones as the base measure, and the amounts and effects of other substances it is mixed with. For example, in many preparations, the kava is combined with other herbal products (e.g., chamomile) that may have similar properties. This would make it even more difficult to differentiate the effects of kava versus the other active ingredients.

Conclusions

Kava appears to be a relatively safe and effective herbal agent for treating everyday anxiety and probably for full-blown anxiety disorders as well. Of course, the major cause for immediate concern with kava use is the reported hepatotoxicity, but concerted efforts are under way in many laboratories and clinical settings to clarify the situation. However, there is almost no sedation when standard doses of up to 240 mg/day kavalactones are used (Singh *et al.*, 1998). Allergic reactions of kava are possible but very rare. Using kava in high doses for prolonged periods may cause a yellow skin rash and skin lesions, although discontinuing or drastically reducing intake rapidly reverses these conditions. However, it should be noted that daily kava use at a dose of 210 mg kavalactones for six months did not cause skin rash or skin lesions in one well-controlled study (Volz and Kieser, 1997). Caution is advised when using kava with benzodiazepines, and medical opinion should be sought before combining these two drugs. Further, if a benzodiazepine is to be tapered, pairing it with kava during the tapering period will decrease the withdrawal effects typically associated with the benzodiazepines (Malsch and Kieser, 2001). In general, when compared to benzodiazepines and alcohol, kava compares most favorably in terms of risk for abuse and addiction.

References

Almeida, J.C. and Grimsley, E.W. (1996) Coma from the health food store: Interaction between kava and alprazolam (letter). *Annals of Internal Medicine*, 125, 940–941.

American Psychiatric Association (1994) *Diagnostic and Statistical Manual of Mental Disorders* (4th ed.), American Psychiatric Association, Washington DC.

Barnett, S.D., Connor, K.M. and Davidson, J.R.T. (2001) The Self Assessment of Reliance and Anxiety (SARA): psychometric properties. *CNS Spectrums*, 6, 854–857.

Bhate, H., Gerster, G. and Gracza, E. (1989) Orale Pramedikation mit Zubereitungen aus *Piper methysticum* bei Operativen Eingriffen in Epiduralanasthesie [in German]. *Erfahrungsheilkunde*, 6, 339–345.

Blumenthal, M. (2002) Kava safety questioned due to case reports of liver toxicity. *HerbalGram*, 55, 26–32.

Boerner, R.J. (2001) Kava kava in the treatment of generalized anxiety disorder, simple phobia and specific social phobia. *Phytotherapy Research*, 15, 646–647.

Bond, A.J. (1998) Drug-induced behavioural disinhibition. Incidence, mechanisms, and therapeutic implications. *CNS Drugs*, 9, 41–57.

Boonen, G. and Haberlein, H. (1998) Influence of genuine kavapyrone enantiomers on the $GABA_A$ binding site. *Planta Medica*, 64(6), 504–506.

Brauer, R.B., Pfab, R. and Becker, K. (2002) Fulminantes Leberversagen nach Einnahme des Pflanzlichen Heilmittels Kava-Kava [in German]. *Zeitschrift fur Gastroenterologie*, 39, 491(P30).

Callaway, E. (1983) The pharmacology of human information processing. *Psychophysiology*, 20, 359–370.

Cawte, J. (1985) Psychoactive substances of the South Seas: betel, kava and pituri. *Australia and New Zealand Journal of Psychiatry*, 19, 83–87.

Connor, K.M. and Davidson, J.R.T. (2002) A placebo-controlled study of kava kava in generalized anxiety disorder. *International Clinical Psychopharmacology*, 17, 185–188.

Cropley, M., Cave, Z., Ellis, J. and Middleton, R.W. (2002) Effect of kava and valerian on human physiological and psychological and psychological responses to mental stress assessed under laboratory conditions. *Phytotherapy Research*, 16, 23–27.

Davies, L.P., Drew, C.A., Duffield, P., Johnson, G.A. and Jamieson, D.D. (1992) Kava pyrones and resin: Studies on $GABA_A$, $GABA_B$ and benzodiazepine binding sites in rodent brain. *Pharmacology and Toxicology*, 71, 120–126.

De Leo, V., La Marca, A., Lanzetta, D., Palazzi, S., Torricelli, M., Facchini, C., *et al.* (2000) Assessment of the association of kava-kava extract and hormone replacement therapy in the treatment of postmenopausal anxiety [original in Italian]. *Minerva Ginecol.*, 52, 263–267.

Denham, A., McIntyre, M. and Whitehouse, J. (2002) Kava – the unfolding story: report on a work-in-progress. *Journal of Alternative and Complementary Medicine*, 8, 237–263.

Derogatis, L.R. (1994) SCL-90, Brief Symptom Inventory and matching clinical rating scales. In M. Maruish (ed.), *Psychological Testing, Treatment Planning, and Outcome Assessment*, Erlbaum, New York.

Ellis, W. (1828) *Polynesian Researches*. Fisher and Jackson, London, vol. 1, pp. 229–231.

Emser, W. and Bartylla, K. (1991) Verbesserung der Schlafqualität. Zur Wirkung von Kava-Extrakt WS 1490 auf das Schlafmuster bei Gesunden [in German]. *TW Neurol. Psychiatr.*, 5, 636–642.

Escher, M., Desmeules, J., Giostra, J. and Mentha, G. (2001) Hepatitis associated with kava, a herbal remedy for anxiety. *British Medical Journal*, 322, 139.

Foo, H. and Lemon, J. (1997) Acute effects of kava, alone or in combination with alcohol, on subjective measures of impairment and intoxication and on cognitive performance. *Drug and Alcohol Review*, 16, 147–155.

Frater, A.S. (1958) Medical aspects of yaqona. *Transactions and Proceedings of Fiji Society*, 5, 31–39.

Gajdusek, D.C. (1979) Recent observations on the use of kava in the New Hebrides. In D.M. Efron, B. Holmstedt, and N.S. Kline (eds), *Ethnopharmacologic Search for Psychoactive Drugs*, Raven Press, New York, pp. 119–125.

Garner, L.F. and Klinger, J.D. (1985) Some visual effects caused by the beverage kava. *Journal of Ethnopharmacology*, 13, 307–311.

Gessner, B. and Cnota, P. (1994) Untersuchung der Vigilan nach Application von Kava-Kava-Extrakt, Diazepam oder Plazebo [in German]. *Zeitschrift fur Phytotherapie*, 15, 30–37.

Gifford, E.W. (1924) *Tongan Myths and Tales*. Bulletin No. 8, Bernice P. Bishop Museum Press, Honolulu, pp. 71–72.

Goodyer, I.N. (1990) Family relationships, life events and childhood psychopathology. *Journal of Child Psychology and Psychiatry*, 31, 161–192.

Greene, R.L. (1980) *The MMPI: An Interpretative Manual*, Grune and Stratton, Orlando, FL.

Hagemann U. (2001) *Pharmaceutical Products Containing Kava-Kava (Piper methysticum) and Kavain, Including Homeopathic Preparations with a Final Concentration up to D6*, German Federal Institute for Drugs and Medical Devices (BfArM), Berlin, November 8.

Hamilton, M. (1959) The assessment of anxiety states by rating. *British Journal of Medical Psychology*, **32**, 50–55.

Heinze, H.J., Münte, T.F., Matzke, M. and Steitz, J. (1994) Pharmacopsychological effects of exazepam and kava-extract in a visual search paradigm assessed with event-related potentials. *Pharmacopsychiatry*, **27**, 224–230.

Hellwig, B. (2000) Lösen Lava-Kava Präparate Leberschäden aus? *Deutsche Apotheker Zeitung*, **29**, 43–48.

Herberg, K.W. (1993) Zum Einfluss von Kava-Spezialextrakt WS 1490 in Kombination mit Ethylalkohol auf Sicherheitsrelevante Leistungsparameter [in German]. *Blutalkohol*, **30**, 96–105.

Herberg, K.W. (1996) Safety-related performance after intake of kava-extract, bromazepam and their combination. *Z. Allgemein Medizinische*, **72**, 973–977.

Hocart, A.M. (1929) *Lau Islands, Fiji.* Bulletin No. 62, Bernice P. Bishop Museum Press, Honolulu, pp. 59–70.

Hoffman, R. and Winter, R. (1996) Therapeutische Möglichkeiten mit Kava Kava bei Angsterkrankungen [in German]. *Psycho Zeitschift Praxis Klin.* **22**, 51–53.

Hunt, E. (1978) Mechanics of verbal ability. *Psychological Review*, **85**, 109–130.

Jamieson, D.D. and Duffield, P.H. (1990) Positive interaction of ethanol and kava resin in mice. *Clinical and Experimental Pharmacology and Physiology*, **17**, 509–514.

Kinzler, E., Krömer, J. and Lehmann, E. (1991) Wirksamkeit Eines Kava-Spezial-Extraktes bei Patienten mit Angst-, Spannungs-, unt Erregungszuständen Nicht-Psychotischer Genese: Doppelblind-Studie Gegen Plazebo über 4 Wochen [in German]. *Arzneimittelforschung*, **41**, 584–588.

Kraft, M., Spahn, T.W., Menzel, J., Senninger, N., Dietl, K.H., Herbst, H., *et al.* (2001) Fulminantes Leberversagen nach Einnahme des pflanzlichen Antidepressivums Kava-Kava [in German]. *Deutsche Medizinische Wochenschrift*, **126**, 970–972.

Lebot, V. (1991) Kava (*Piper methysticum* Forst f.). The Polynesian dispersal of an Oceania plant. In P.A. Cox and S.A. Bannack, (eds.), *Islands, Plants and Polynesians: An Introduction to Polynesian Ethnobotany*, Dioscorides Press, Portland, OR, pp. 169–201.

Lebot, V. and Cabalion, P. (1988) *Kavas of Vanuatu: Cultivars of* Piper methysticum *Forst.* Technical Paper No. 195, South Pacific Commission, Noumea.

Lebot, V. and Lévesque, J. (1989) The origin and distribution of kava (*Piper methysticum*). A phytochemical approach. *Allertonia*, **5**(2), 223–281.

Lebot, V. and Lévesque, J. (1996) Genetic control of kavalactone chemotypes in *Piper methysticum* cultivars. *Phytochemistry*, **43**, 397–403.

Lebot, V., Merlin, M. and Lindstrom, L. (1997) *Kava: The Pacific Elixir*, Healing Arts Press, Rochester, VT.

Lehmann, E., Klieser, E., Klimke, A., Krach, H. and Spatz, R. (1989) The efficacy of cavain in patients suffering from anxiety. *Pharmacopsychiatry*, **22**, 258–262.

Lehmann, E., Kinzler, E. and Friedemann, J. (1996) Efficacy of a special kava extract (*Piper methysticum*) in patients with states of anxiety, tension and excitedness of non-mental origin: A double-blind placebo-controlled study of four weeks treatment. *Phytomedicine*, **3**, 113–119.

Lemert, E.M. (1967) Secular use of kava in Tonga. *Quarterly Journal of Studies on Alcohol*, **28**, 328–341.

Lewin, L. (1886) *Über* Piper methysticum *(kawa-kawa)*, Medical Society, Berlin.

Lindenberg, Von D. and Pitule-Schödel, H. (1990) D, L-Kavain im Vergleich zu Oxazepam bei Angstzustanden [in German]. *Fortschritte Medizinische*, **108**, 49–54.

Malsch, U. and Kieser, M. (2001) Efficacy of kava-kava in the treatment of non-psychotic anxiety, following pretreatment with benzodiazepines. *Psychopharmacology (Berlin)*, **157**, 277–283.

Mathews, J.D., Riley, M.D., Fejo, L., Munoz, E., Milns, N.R., Gardner, I.D., *et al.* (1988) Effects of the heavy usage of kava on physical health: Summary of a pilot study in an Aboriginal community. *Medical Journal of Australia*, **148**, 548–555.

Mathews, J.M., Etheridge, A.S. and Black, S.R. (2002) Inhibition of human cytochrome P450 activities by kava extract and kavalactones. *Drug Metabolism and Disposition*, **30**, 1153–1157.

Meyer, H.J. (1979) Pharmacology of kava. In D.M. Efron, B. Holmstedt, and N.S. Kline (eds), *Ethnopharmacologic Search for Psychoactive Drugs*, Raven Press, New York, pp. 133–140.

MMWR (2002) Hepatic toxicity possibly associated with kava-containing products – United States, Germany, and Switzerland, 1999–2002. *Morbidity and Mortality Weekly Report*. Centers for Disease Control and Prevention, Atlanta, GA, 51(47), 1065–1067.

Möller, H.J. and Heuberger, M.L. (1989) Anxiolytische potenz von D, L-Kavain [in German]. *Münchener Medizinische Wochenschrift* 131, 656–659.

Morrison, J. (1935) *The Journals of James Morrison*. Golden Cockerel Press, London, p. 151.

Münte, T.F., Heinze, H.J., Matzke, M. and Steitz, J. (1993) Effects of oxazepam and an extract of kava roots (*Piper methysticum*) on event-related potentials in a word recognition task. *Neuropsychobiology*, 27, 46–53.

Neuhaus, W., Ghaemi, Y., Schmidt, T. and Lehmann, E. (2000) Treatment of perioperative anxiety in suspected breast carcinoma with a phytogenic tranquilizer. *Zentralbl Gynakol.*, 11, 561–565.

NIMH (1970) National Institutes of Mental Health. 12-CGI. Clinical Global Impressions. In Guy, W. and Bonato, R. (eds), *Manual for the ECDEU Assessment Battery*. 2 Rev. Ed, Chevy Chase, Maryland.

Norton, S.A. and Ruze, P. (1994) Kava dermopathy. *Journal of the American Academy of Dermatology*, 31, 89–97.

Pfeiffer, C.C., Murphree, H.B. and Goldstein, L. (1979) Effect of kava in normal subjects and patients. In D.H. Efron, B. Holmstedt and N.S. Kline (eds), *Ethnopharmacologic Search for Psychoactive Drugs*, Raven Press, New York, pp. 155–161.

Poolsup, N., Po, L. and Knight, T. (2000) Pharmacogenetics and psychopharmacotherapy. *Journal of Clinical Pharmacology and Therapeutics*, 25, 197–220.

Posner, M.I. (1978) *Chronometric Explorations of Mind*. Hillsdale, NJ: Erlbaum.

Prescott, J., Jamieson, D., Emdur, N. and Duffield, P. (1993) Acute effects of kava on measures of cognitive performance, physiological function and mood. *Drug and Alcohol Review*, 12, 49–58.

Prescott, J. and McCall, G. (1988) *Kava: Use and Abuse in Australia and the South Pacific*. National Drug and Alcohol Research Center, University of New South Wales, Kensington, Australia.

Reuters (2002) Britain to ban kava herbal medicines, *www.reuters.com*. Accessed December 23, 2002.

Russell, P.N., Bakker, D. and Singh, N.N. (1987) The effects of kava on alerting and speed of access of information from long-term memory. *Bulletin of the Psychonomic Society*, 25, 236–237.

Russmann, S., Lauterburg, B.H. and Helbling, A. (2001) Kava hepatotoxicity. *Annals of Internal Medicine*, 135, 68–69.

Ruze, P. (1990) Kava-induced dermopathy: A niacin deficiency? *Lancet*, 335, 1442–1445.

Sass, M., Schnabel, S. and Kröger, J. (2001) Akutes Leberversgen durch Kava-Kava – eine seltene Indikation zur Lebertransplantation [in German]. *Zeitschrift fur Gastroenterologie*, 39, 491(P29).

Schelosky, L., Raffauf, C., Jendroska, K. and Poewe, W. (1995) Kava and dopamine antagonism (letter). *Journal of Neurology, Neurosurgery and Psychiatry*, 58, 639–640.

Scherer, J. (1998) Kava-kava extract in anxiety disorders: An outpatient observational study. *Advances in Therapy*, 15, 261–269.

Schmidt J. (2001) *Analysis of kava side effects. Reports concerning the liver*. M. Lindenmaier and J. Brinckmann, translators. December 31, 2001 (unpublished). Courtesy: American Herbal Products Association, Silver Springs, MD.

Schmidt, M. and Nahrstedt, A. (2002) Is kava hepatotoxic? [in German]. *Deutsche Apotheker Zeitung*, 142, 1006–1011.

Scholing, W.E. and Clausen, H.D. (1997) über die Wirkung von D, L-Kavain: Erfahrungen mit dem Präparat Neuronika® [in German]. *Medizinische. Klin.*, 72, 1301–1306.

Shulgin, A.T. (1973) The narcotic pepper: The chemistry and pharmacology of *Piper methysticum* and related species. *Bulletin of Narcotics*, 25, 59–74.

Siegel, R.K. (1976) Herbal intoxication. *JAMA*, 23, 473–476.

Siegers, C.P., Honold, E. and Krall, B. (1992) Ergebnisse einer Anwendungsbeobachtung L1090 mit Laitan® Kapseln [in German]. *Arzneimittelforschung*, 39, 7–11.

Singh, N.N. and Beale, I.L. (1986) Behavioral assessment of pharmacotherapy. *Behavior Change*, 3, 34–40.

Singh, N.N., Ellis, C.R. and Singh, Y.N. (1998) A double blind, placebo-controlled study of the effects of kava (Kavatrol®) on daily stress and anxiety in adults. *Alternative Therapies*, 4, 98–99.

Singh, Y.N. (1992) Kava: an Overview. *Journal of Ethnopharmacology*, 37, 13–45.

Singh, Y.N. and Singh, N.N. (2002) Therapeutic potential of kava in the treatment of anxiety disorders. *CNS Drugs*, 16, 731–743.

Staedt, U., Holm, E., Heep, J., Rienmuller, S., Kortsik, C. and Steiner, G. (1991) Zum Wirkungsprofil von d,l-Kavain: Psychometrie, EEG und Fremdbeurteilungsskala [in German]. *Medwelt*, 42, 881–891.

Stoller, R. (2000) Leberschädigungen unter Kava-Extrakten [in German]. *Schweizerische ärztezeitung*, 81, 1335–1336.

Strahl, S., Ehret, V., Dahm, H.H. and Maier, K.P. (1998) Nekrotisierende Hepatitis nach Einnahme pflanzlicher Heilmittel (Necrotizing hepatitis after taking herbal remedies) [in German, English abstract]. *Deutsche Medizinische Wochenschrift*, 123, 1410–1414.

Titcomb, M. (1948) Kava in Hawaii. *Journal of the Polynesian Society*, 57, 105–171.

Toniolo Neto, J. (1999) Tolerability of kava-kava extract WS 1490 on anxiety disorders: Multi-center Brazilian study. *Revista Brasileira de Medicina*, 56, 280–284.

Van Der Bijl, P. and Roelofse, J.A. (1991) Disinhibitory reactions to benzodiazepines: a review. *Journal of Oral and Maxillofacial Surgery*, 49, 519–523.

Volz, H.P. (1996) The anxiolytic efficacy of the kava special extract WS 1490 using long-term therapy. A randomized, double-blind study. *Quarterly Review of Natural Medicine*, Fall issue, 185–186.

Volz, H.P. and Kieser, M. (1997) Kava-kava extract WS 1490 versus placebo in anxiety disorders: A randomized placebo-controlled 25-week outpatient trial. *Pharmacopsychiatry*, 30, 1–5.

von Zersson, D. (1986) Clinical self-rating scales (CSRC) of the Munich psychiatric information system (Psychis München). In N.T. Sartorius and A. Ban (eds), *Assessment of Depression*, Springer, Berlin, pp. 279–303.

Waller, D.P. (2002) *Report on Kava and Liver Damage*, American Herbal Products Association, Silver Springs, Maryland.

Wanwirolmuk, S., Bhawan, S., Coville, P. and Chalcroft, S. (1998) Genetic polymorphism of debrisoquine (CYP2D6) and proguanil (CYP2C19) in South Pacific Polynesian populations. *European Journal of Clinical Pharmacology*, 54, 431–435.

Warnecke, G., Pfaender, H., Gerster, G. and Gracza, E. (1990) Wirksamkeit von Kawa-Kawa Extrakt beim Klimakterischen Syndrom [in German]. *Zeitschrift fur Phytotherapie*, 11, 81–86.

Warnecke, Von, G. (1991) Psychosomatische Dysfunktionen im Weiblichen Klimakterium: Klinische Wirksamkeit und Vertraglichkeit von Kava Extrakt WS 1490 [in German]. *Fortschritte Medizinische*, 109, 119–122.

Werry, J.S. (1998) Anxiolytics and sedatives. In S. Reiss and M.G. Aman (eds), *Psychotropic Medication and Developmental Disabilities: The International Consensus Handbook*, Ohio State University Nisonger Center, Columbus, OH, pp. 201–214.

Wheatley, D. (2001) Kava and valerian in the treatment of stress-induced insomnia. *Phytotherapy Research*, 15, 549–551.

Woelk, H., Kapoula, O., Lehri, S., Schroter, K. and Weinholz, P. (1993) Behandlung von Angst-Patienten Doppelblindstudie: Kava-Spezialextrakt WS 1490 versus Benzodiazepine [in German]. *Ztschr. Allg. Medizinische*, 69, 271–277.

Zepernick, B. (1972) *Arzneipflanzen der Polynesier* [in German], Dietrich Reimer, Berlin.

Zigmond, A.S. and Snaith, R.P. (1983) The Hospital Anxiety and Depression Scale. *Acta Psychiatrica Scandinavica*, 67, 361–370.

Zou, L., Harkey, M.R. and Henderson, G.L. (2002) Effects of herbal components on cDNA-expressed cytochrome P450 enzyme catalytic activity. *Life Sciences*, 71, 1579–1589.

Zung, W.W.K. (1965) A self-rating depression scale. *Archives of General Psychiatry*, 12, 63–70.

Index

adulterants   42
Ahouia   59
alkaloids in kava
   molecular properties of   89–90
Anthracnose   35
anxiety   142–52
   associated with menopause   147–8
   cognitive function   150–2
   disorders and symptomatology
      142–7
   due to medical conditions   148–9
   seizure management   149–50
   sleep and insomnia   149
Ap   60
Apin   59
army worms   36
ava; ava-ava; awa; awa-awa
   see kava

betel nut
   chewing   51
   culture   51
'betel people', the   51
'body' of the kava drink   25
Bogong   59
Borogu   59

Choiseul   53
Cook, James   5, 64
cucumber mosaic virus (CMV)   34

desmethoxyyangonin   85
dieback disease   33–4
7,8-dihydromethysticin   84–5
7,8-dihydroyangonin   94–5
diseases and pests
   bacteria   35–6
   dieback disease   33–4
   fungal diseases   35
   insects and other pests   36
   nematodes   34–5
diversity in kava cultivars   56–60

Fiji islands
   custom in drinking kava in   1–3
   gifting kava   16
   kava production and marketing   45–6
   myths on kava   12–13
   preparation of kava   1, 24–5
   traditional classification system   57
Fiji National Kava Council   40
flavokavins in kava   90–1
Forster   6, 64

Giant African land snail   36
green kava   23

Hawai'i   11
   kava circles   18
   kava custom   52–3
   traditional classification system   60
   traditional religious practices   21
high performance liquid chromatography
      (HPLC)   42–3, 91–2
   in distribution of kavalactones   78
   in ethnobotanical studies   98
   in standardization procedure for
      kavalactones   127
Honolulu   57, 58

INA Methods Validation Program
      (INA MVP)   42
Institute for Nutraceutical Advancement
      (INA)   42
intercropping kava with other plants   32–3

kasa   1, 57–8
kava
   adverse effects   *see* kava – adverse effects
   alkaloids, flavokavins and other
      components   87–91
   bars/circles   *see* kava bars/circles
   botanic origins   14–16, 65–8
   centers of usage   53
   ceremony vs. *soma* (Vedic) ritual   52

kava   (*Continued*)
  chewing, origin of   24–5
  clinical studies   142–52
  cloning of   29, 50
  contemporary distribution   11
  cultivar names   56–60
  cultivation   *see* kava cultivation
  culture   51
  current clinical uses   141
  different interpretations on kava drinking   5–7
  distribution of chemotypes   69–72
  etymology of   55–60
  geographical distribution of   10, 50–5
  as a gift   16–19
  historical uses   140
  inhibitions to the development of
    micropropagation system   30–1
  interaction between isozyme and chemotype
    of   72–3
  interaction of environment, ontogeny and
    chemotypes of   68–9
  'kava people', the   51
  maceration methods of   24–7
  medicinal uses of   22–3
  methods of kava preparation and
    consumption   23–7
  morphological features   57
  myths in kava-using societies   *see also* Fiji
    islands; Vanuatu; Tanna; Papua
  origin of   51–5
  plant morphology   60–4
  political functions   19
  psychoactive chemicals   1, 42, 57, 72–3,
    96, 152
  role of kava as a cash crop   43–8
  taxonomy and nomenclature   64–5
  traditional religious uses of   20–2
  utensils used in kava preparation   24
kava – adverse effects   152–7
  drug interactions   155–7
  hepatotoxicity   130, 154–5
  physical and cutaneous effects   152–4
  quality of research evidence   157–9
  tolerability surveillance   152
  visual effects   154
kava bars/circles
  Melanesian   *see nakamal*
  Polynesian   18
kava cultivation
  constraints   *see also* diseases and pests
  crop care   33
  cropping   32–3
  direct planting   31
  false kava species   31
  harvesting   36–7
  in vivo propagation   30–1
  nurseries and transplanting   31–2

  planting material   30
  processing   *see also* processing kava
  site selection   29–30
kava micropropagation system   30–1
kava weevil borer   36
kavain   1, 7, 43, 69–71, 76–80, 85, 87, 88,
    89, 93, 94–5, 96, 97–8, 104, 105, 106,
    107–8, 110, 111–27, 144, 145, 148,
    150, 152, 157
  and 7, 8-dihydrokavain   85
kavalactones in kava   1, 11, 22, 26, 41, 76
  analytical techniques for the isolation and
    purification of   91–3
  early studies on   104–6
  INA MVP procedure for   43
  metabolism and elimination in animals   94–5
  metabolism and elimination in humans   95–6
  molecular properties of   87–9
  pharmacodynamic studies on   *see*
    pharmacodynamic studies
  pharmacological mechanisms of action   *see*
    pharmacological mechanisms of action
  physicochemical and pharmacokinetic properties
    of   93–6
  stability of   93
  standardization procedure for kavalactones   127
  structure elucidation of   79–87
  structure–activity relationships (SAR)
    of   96–7
  toxicity effects   *see* toxicity studies of kava
  ultraviolet-visible and infrared spectra of
    88–9
  see also yangonin; methysticin;
    7,8-dihydromethysticin; kavain;
    desmethoxyyangonin
kavapyrones   *see* kavalactones
kawain   *see* kavain

lewena   1, 58
Liwa   60
loa kasa balavu   57
loa kasa leka   58

Makea   60
Malmalbo   59
marketing and economics
  role of kava as a cash crop   43–7
  trading systems and networks   43–4
mealy bugs   36
Melanesia   3, 4, 10, 14, 18, 50, 51, 54, 56,
    65, 69, 157
Melmel   59
methysticin   82–5, 94
Micronesia   3, 4, 10, 14, 15, 19, 40, 52,
    54, 69, 80, 132
mites   36
Mo'i   60

nakamal 18
    preparation of kava 25
Natural History Museum (London) 5

Oceania 3, 50, 51–2, 55, 64, 76, 140
    cultural traditions in 51
    importance of kava in 5

Pacific Island Kava Council 40
papa 60
Papua New Guinea
    gifting kava 17
    myths on kava 14
    preparation of kava 25
Pentecost islands
    chemotypic diversity of kava 69–72
    myths on kava 12
    traditional classification system 58–9
pharmacodynamic studies
    analgesia and local anesthetic effects
        107–8
    anesthesia and sedation 106
    anticonvulsant actions 114–15
    information processing and cognition
        111–14
    muscle paralyzing actions 108–10
    neuroprotection 115–16
    studies on other effects 116–17
    visual effects 110–11
pharmacological mechanisms of action
    effects on GABA and benzodiazepine
        receptors 122–4
    effects on ion channels 117–22
    effects on monoamine uptake carriers 124
    effects on neurotransmitters 125
Pia 59
Piper aduncum 31, 67
Piper auritum 31, 67
Piper methysticum *see* kava
Piper wickmannii 65–73
Pohnpei
    gifting kava 16
    preparation of kava 25
Pohnpei kava 25
polybags *see* polypots
Polynesia 3, 4, 7, 10, 11, 14, 15, 17, 18,
        20, 30, 50, 51–6, 58, 60, 65, 67, 69,
        71, 80, 132, 157
    preparation of kava 24–5, 26–7
polypots 32
processing kava
    cutting, peeling and sorting 37
    drying 38
    industrial processing 39–40
    powdering 39
    storage 38–9
    washing 37

qila balavu 58
quality measures taken by the governments 40–3
    adulterants 41–2
    quality control 40
    quality markers of kava 42
    specifications 41
    typical HPLC methods 42–3

reniform nematodes 35
Rhowen 59
root-knot nematodes 35
roots and rootlets, lateral *see waka*
    see also lewena; kasa
rootstock 76

Scholander, Daniel 5
Sclerotium rolfsii 35
Secretariat of the Pacific Community (SPC) 40
'shadow' of the kava drink 25
Sphaerulina leaf spots 35
spiral nematodes 34
'spirit' of the kava drink *see* 'shadow' of the
    kava drink

Tahiti 69, 113, 140, 151
    kava drinking in 54
    traditional classification system 60
Tanna
    gifting kava 16–17
    myths on kava 13
    preparation of kava 25, 26–7
    traditional classification system 58–9
Tonga
    traditional classification 58
toxicity studies of kava 127–33
    carcinogenicity 132
    cutaneous effects 128–30
    hepatotoxicity 130
    interactions with other substances 130–2
    mutagenicity and teratogenicity 132
    precautions and contraindications 133
    tolerance and addiction potential 132
transplanting kava plants 32

Vanuatu
    cultivar classification system 58
    gifting kava 17
    kava production and marketing 45–6
    kava usage 53
    myths on kava 12
    preparation of kava 25
vula kasa leka 57

waka 1, 58

yangonin 79–82, 95
yaqona *see* kava

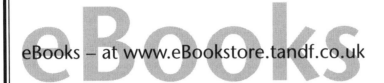

Printed and bound by CPI Group (UK) Ltd, Croydon, CR0 4YY

30/10/2024

01781168-0001